CATARACT SURGERY

A Patient's Guide to Treatment

Second Edition

Robert K. Maloney, M.D., M.A. (Oxon)
Neda Shamie, M.D.

D1005395

Addicus Books
Omaha, Nebraska

An Addicus Nonfiction Book

ISBN: 978-1-950091-38-6
Illustrations by JIREHDESIGN.com
Cover design by Ryan Delaney and Jack Kusler
Interior design by Jack Kusler

This book is not intended to serve as a substitute for a physician. Nor is it the authors' intent to give medical advice contrary to that of an attending physician.

Library of Congress Cataloging-in-Publication Data

Names: Maloney, Robert K., author. | Shamie, Neda, author.
Title: Cataract surgery : a patient's guide to treatment / Robert K. Maloney, M.D., M.A. (Oxon), Neda Shamie, M.D.
Description: Second edition. | Omaha, Nebraska : Addicus Books, 2020. | Includes index. |
Identifiers: LCCN 2020009730 (print) | LCCN 2020009731 (ebook) | ISBN 9781950091386 (trade paperback) | ISBN 9781950091409 (pdf) | ISBN 9781950091416 (epub) | ISBN 9781950091423 (kindle edition)
Subjects: LCSH: Cataract—Surgery—Popular works.
Classification: LCC RE451 .M33 2020 (print) | LCC RE451 (ebook) | DDC | 617.7/42059—dc23
LC record available at https://lccn.loc.gov/2020009730
LC ebook record available at https://lccn.loc.gov/2020009731

Addicus Books, Inc.
P.O. Box 45327
Omaha, Nebraska 68145
www.AddicusBooks.com

Printed in the United States of America
10 9 8 7 6 5 4 3 2 1

*To the thousands of patients who have trusted us
with their most precious sense—their sight*

Contents

Acknowledgments

I wish to thank my father, who taught me to be uncompromising in the pursuit of excellence, and my mother, who taught me that great relationships require compromise. I particularly thank my fabulous wife, Nicole, for her patience with the demands of my chosen career. At times, she must wish that I had listened more to my mother's advice.

—*Robert K. Maloney, M.D.*

I wish to thank my husband and my daughters without whose support I could not nurture my love of my chosen field. Their support allows me to maintain balance in my life and brings color and fulfillment to my days.

—*Neda Shamie, M.D.*

Introduction

Of all the amazing components of the human anatomy, the eyes may be the most marvelous. They are your primary tools of awareness. The ability to see allows you independence, mobility, and appreciation of visual beauty and form.

If your vision is starting to blur and you think you might have cataracts, put your mind at ease. Cataracts are usually painless and are not harmful to other parts of your eyes. They are not a sign of disease, nor are they "growths." They are simply a clouding of the lens of the eye. In most cases, cataracts are as normal a part of aging as the "silver threads among the gold" (in the words of an old song) that appear when your hair begins to gray.

Cataracts develop so gradually that you probably won't need any treatment for them at first. A stronger eyeglass prescription will likely help in the early stages. Eventually, your vision will become blurrier, some things will seem out of focus, and you'll need new prescriptions more often. Objects might appear yellowish. Glare or halos from light sources could make night driving difficult. You might have trouble reading, both close up and at a distance—fine print in a book, for example, and street signs along the highway. When these symptoms interfere with your day-to-day activities, you may want to consider surgery.

By age sixty-five, most Americans have early-stage cataracts, and, by age eighty, most have had cataract surgery. Surgeons perform some 3 million cataract operations a year in the United States, with a very high success rate and few complications. We are fortunate to live in a time and a place where outpatient surgery, which takes just minutes, can painlessly replace a clouded natural lens with a state-of-the-art synthetic lens. Within a day or two of your surgery, you'll marvel at how clear and vivid your world has become.

In the United States, cataract surgery is among the most effective and safest surgical procedures performed—especially in the hands of a highly qualified and experienced eye surgeon. Replacement lenses do an excellent job of restoring vision (with or without glasses, depending on the type of lens implanted). Recovery is rapid—you can resume most of your normal activities within a few days.

This book describes how the healthy eye functions, how cataracts can interfere with clear eyesight, and how clarity can be restored. It explains all your options if cataracts are starting to cloud your vision. It can help you and your doctor determine the right time for surgery.

You, or someone you care about, might find great reassurance in the knowledge that cataracts can be safely and successfully treated and that, after they are removed, cataracts do not return. Advances in cataract surgery have made it possible for millions of people to enjoy the independence and the aesthetic pleasure of clear vision for decades beyond what was once possible.

The Human Eye and How It Works

To understand how cataracts cause blurry vision, you may find it helpful to learn about the structure of the eye and how it works. The eye is a complex organ that performs many complicated functions in a very short time—in the blink of an eye, one might say.

Anatomy of the Eye

If you could examine an entire human eye, you'd see a sphere about an inch in diameter—the size of a large gumball. The eyeball itself is really three thin layers of tissue that surround a fluid-filled center.

Sclera

The outside layer is the "white of the eye," called the *sclera*. It is the tough, opaque tissue that serves as the eye's structural outer layer. Six tiny muscles connect to it around the eye and control the eye's movements. The *optic nerve* carries the visual image from the eye to the brain.

Cornea

Curving out from the sclera, the clear *cornea* is the "front window" of the eye. It is the first layer through which light enters the eye. The cornea is tough and protects the inside of your eye from dust

Eye Anatomy

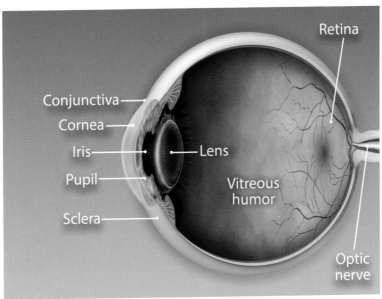

The different parts of the eye.

and germs. Packed with nerve fibers, it is also quite sensitive to pain. This pain sensitivity is one of the cornea's protective qualities, signaling tearing or a brisk blink to wash out a grain of sand.

Iris

Behind the clear cornea is a thin layer of colored tissue, called the *iris*. When we say that someone's eyes are blue, brown, or green, we are talking about the color of the iris. Besides being an expressive feature of the face, the iris is essential to clear vision. It surrounds the round, black *pupil*. It is through the pupil that light enters the eye and allows us to see.

Lens

The *lens* focuses light entering the eye so we can see clearly, just as a camera lens focuses light

Normal Eye

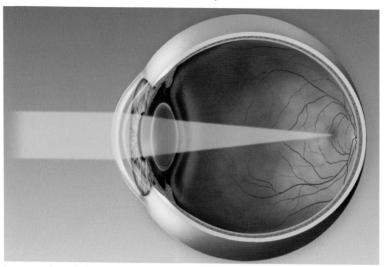

In a normal eye, light passes through the lens and focuses on the retina. Vision is sharp.

Eye with Cataract

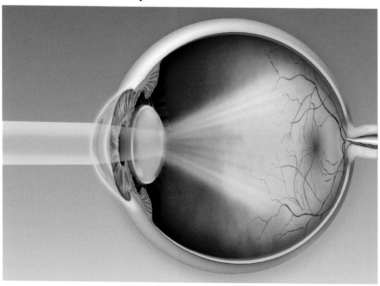

A cataract has formed in the lens of the eye, causing the light rays to scatter rather than focus on the retina. Vision is blurry.

entering the camera to create a clear photo. The lens sits behind the iris and pupil. It is surrounded by a tiny muscle that allows it to change shape, so that it can focus across a full range of distances.

There are three distinct layers in the lens, sometimes compared to the layers of a peach: The *capsular bag* or *capsule* (the peach "skin") is a thin, clear membrane that forms the outside layer of the lens. The *cortex* (comparable to the peach "flesh") is the soft, clear material just beneath the capsular bag. The *nucleus* (the "pit" of the peach) is the firm center, or core of the lens.

Retina

The *retina* is the "screen" located at the back of the eye onto which light rays entering the eye are focused. Specialized cells within the retina convert the light to electrical signals that flow through the optic nerve to the brain. The *macula* is the focal point at the center of the retina. Within the macula are millions of light-sensitive nerve endings that act as *photoreceptors*. The photoreceptors called *rods* are sensitive to brightness and allow us to see in dim light. The photoreceptors called *cones* respond to the varying wavelengths of light that produce different colors.

Features That Protect the Eyes

The eyeballs are protected, in part, by their location—they are embedded in sockets, which are strongholds of bone, fat, and muscle. Other protective features of the eye are:

- *Eyelashes*—which protect your eyes from dust, contaminants, and other small particles.

- *Eyebrows*—which trap liquids (such as perspiration) and particles that might otherwise find their way into your eyes.
- *Tears*—which supply moisture that not only keeps your eyes from drying out but also contain substances that fight bacteria. If a foreign object gets into your eye, tear production increases to flush it out.
- *Eyelids*—which work like windshield wipers when you blink, to spread tears across the cornea. Blinking is usually automatic—you seldom have to remember to blink—but it is also a protective reflex that goes into action when your eyes perceive an object moving toward them or are assaulted by extremely bright light.

How Vision Occurs

It might be helpful to think of seeing as four distinct processes, which are roughly similar to the way a camera processes an image.

Light Reflects off an Object

Suppose you are on a tropical beach, looking at a palm tree as its fronds wave in the ocean breeze. You're actually seeing the light from the sun reflecting off the leaves—just as a photograph is an image of light reflecting off an object. If this were not the case, then you'd be able to see objects at night, or photograph them just as well as in daylight.

Light Enters the Eye

As light reaches the eye, it first enters the clear, curved cornea. The curved surface of the cornea bends the incoming light as it enters the eye so that the rays begin to converge instead of remaining parallel.

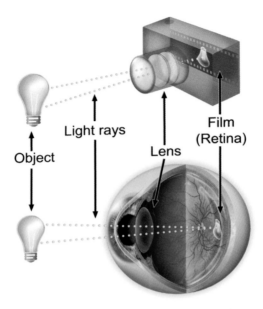

Light passes through the eye's lens and focuses on the retina in the same way that light passes through a camera lens and onto the film.

Thus, the cornea begins the work of focusing light in the eye.

After passing through the cornea, light is bathed in a thin layer of liquid, the *aqueous humor,* before it reaches the iris. The pupil contracts or expands (dilates) to regulate the amount of light allowed into the eye's interior. When you walk out of a dark movie theater into bright daylight, you've probably experienced that "blinding" sensation before the iris has time to contract, adjusting to the difference in light.

Light Is Focused in the Lens

The lens, by changing its shape, also contributes to the eye's focusing work. The lens is a round disc with one side flatter than the other. When you were younger, most likely your lens was perfectly clear

Myopia (Nearsighted Vision)

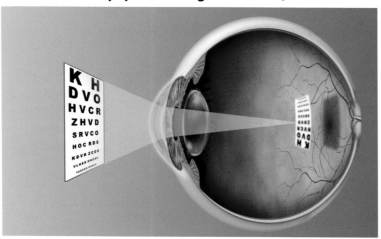

The focusing power of the cornea and lens is too strong, so light from an object is focused in front of the retina. The result is blurry vision.

and quite flexible. The lens is like a small, clear gelcap with a thin but sturdy exterior. If you squeeze a gelcap in the middle, it gets thinner and flatter; if you squeeze the ends, it gets thicker and more rounded. That's basically what happens to the eye's natural lens when you focus on objects at varying distances, except that the work of "squeezing," or contracting, is done by a muscle called the *ciliary muscle* and the ligament attached to it, the *zonule*. This muscle and ligament also hold the lens in place.

When you focus on something close up, the ciliary muscles contract, making the lens thicker and rounder. As your focus moves outward to more-distant objects, the muscles relax and the lens becomes thinner and flatter. Thus, the normal lens projects a clear image onto the retina, at the back of the eye, whether the source of the image is near or far, or somewhere between. This shape-changing adjustment to distance is called *accommodation*. Although

Hyperopia (Farsighted Vision)

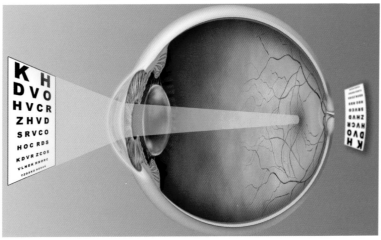

The focusing power of the cornea and lens is too weak. Light from an object is focused behind the retina, causing blurry vision.

the cornea does the initial focusing, it is the lens and its accommodation ability that allow you to focus well at different distances.

Light Signals Are Interpreted by the Brain

After passing through the lens, the light passes through a spacious cavity behind the lens. Finally, the light reaches its destination—the retina, which receives images in much the same way that camera film does. After the retina's specialized cells, rods, and cones have converted the image to signals that the brain can understand, the signals are finally carried to the brain through the nerve bundle at the back of the eye—the optic nerve, which consists of millions of nerve fibers. The brain receives and interprets the signals, and it is at that point that we actually see. Vision occurs only when an image reaches the brain and is identified.

The eye is sometimes described as an extension of the brain, and if there is severe damage to the optic nerve or the image-processing centers of the brain, the eye loses its ability to "see."

Eye Structure Abnormalities

The process described above works best if the eye is a perfect sphere and the cornea is smooth and rounded. Often this isn't the case. The eye might be shorter or longer from front to back than it is from top to bottom, or the cornea's curvature might be irregular or asymmetric.

Farsightedness and Nearsightedness

If the length of your eyes is shorter than normal from front to back, then you have *hyperopia,* or *farsightedness,* and you see distant objects more clearly than near ones. If the opposite is true—if your eyes are longer than normal from front to back— you have *myopia,* or *nearsightedness,* and you have trouble seeing distant objects.

Astigmatism

The cornea's curvature should be rounded, like the side of a basketball. If, instead, it's shaped more like the side of a football, it will produce two focal points instead of just one. This condition is called *astigmatism* and it causes blurring and distortion, especially up close.

Cataracts and Lens Function

You can see how many structures and processes are important to the act of seeing. If just one structure is defective, or one process doesn't work properly, the eyesight—so important to almost everything we do—can be greatly damaged. Like other parts of our bodies, our eyes don't function as well when we age as they did when we were young.

Cataracts are the most common age-related eye defect. The next chapter will explain what cataracts are and how they interfere with the intricate function of the eyes.

2

What Is a Cataract?

If you're in your midfifties or older, there's a good chance that your eyes have started to develop cataracts. You can't see them, you can't feel them, and until they begin to affect your vision, you don't really need to do anything about them except continue to take good care of your eyes. That means having regular eye exams and protecting your eyes—from injury, from the sun's *ultraviolet (UV) rays,* and from irritants such as dust and wind.

A cataract is a clouding of the natural lens inside the eye. The clouded areas are often called *opacities* because they are opaque, and light cannot pass through them. The lens must be crystal clear to focus light well, and so the areas of opacity interfere with good vision.

How Do Cataracts Form?

Protein fibers in the lens, called *crystallines,* are precisely arranged in thousands of layers. Usually because of aging, the proteins deteriorate or become "disarranged." Some scientists believe that these fragmented proteins cause the "clumps" that cloud areas of the lens. These dense areas are cataracts, and as they become larger they cause noticeable vision loss.

Normal Eye

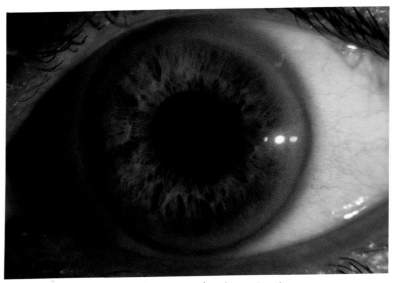

Normal eye. The pupil appears black because there is no cataract.

People sometimes confuse cataracts with an unrelated lens condition, *presbyopia*—a stiffening of the lens also caused by aging. Throughout life, the lens continues to manufacture new layers of cells, and the accumulation of layers makes the lens less pliable. As the lens loses its flexibility, it also loses the ability to adjust its focus from far to near as well as it once could. Around age forty-five most people—even those who have always had excellent vision—find that, figuratively speaking, their arms are "too short." They have to hold books and magazines farther from their eyes in order to focus on the print. If loss of reading vision is your only problem, you can probably solve it with inexpensive reading glasses.

Chapter 4 discusses the causes of cataracts in further detail.

How Common Are Cataracts?

Nearly everyone will eventually have cataracts. Estimates differ because not all who are affected seek treatment, but current research indicates that by age seventy-five at least 70 percent of Americans either cannot see well because of cataracts or have already had cataract surgery. You'll likely notice the beginnings of cataract-related vision problems in your early to midsixties.

Cataract surgery is the most common surgical procedure in the United States. Some 3 million Americans have cataract surgery every year, often in an outpatient procedure that takes less than fifteen minutes. The surgeon replaces the clouded natural lens with a clear synthetic lens through a tiny incision. These procedures nearly always succeed in greatly improving the patient's vision, with almost no interruption in daily activities.

How Do Cataracts Affect Vision?

As explained earlier, all light entering the eye passes through the lens. Your lens must be clear for light to focus properly on the retina. Therefore, any clouding of the lens will affect your vision to some extent.

In most people, cataracts develop gradually, and their eyesight may be adequate for several years before surgery is necessary. Other people experience more rapid progression of cataracts, especially if several areas of the lens are affected. Cataracts that form directly behind the pupil are likely to cause problems sooner than cataracts closer to the edges of the lens.

As more and more of the lens becomes opaque, the clouded areas scatter the light that enters and

Nuclear Cataract

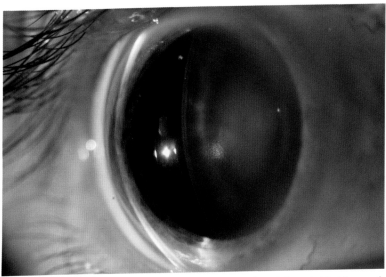

A nuclear cataract is visable in this eye as a cloudy, yellowish oval shape behind the pupil.

prevent it from focusing properly on the retina. If you have cataracts, blurry vision might make it hard to drive at night. You might see glare or halos around lights. Your vision might be blurred or hazy—like trying to see through a waterfall. Eventually, the lens takes on a yellow or brown tinge, which affects your ability to distinguish colors, particularly shades of purple and blue.

Again, these changes might occur so slowly that you don't notice them until someone points out that your socks don't match! Unless they are persistently ignored and become hypermature, cataracts do not cause discomfort—itching, burning, or aching—nor a discharge from your eye, nor do they create redness, swelling, or inflammation. If you have symptoms

Cortical Cataract

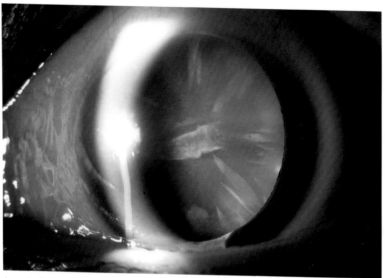

A cortical cataract appears as whitish spokes extending into the center of the pupil.

such as these, see your eye doctor to find out what is causing them.

Types of Cataracts

You will usually see cataracts classified according to their location on the lens: nuclear, cortical, or subcapsular. A nuclear cataract is the most common and is the type most associated with aging, although older patients often have more than one type.

Nuclear Cataracts

A *nuclear cataract,* as the name suggests, is a clouding of the center of the lens, almost always due to aging. One of the early symptoms, oddly enough, is that your near vision will improve for a while. This improvement, referred to as *second sight,* is short-lived, as the cataract becomes increasingly dense,

Subcapsular Cataract

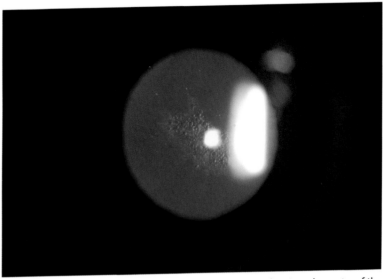

A posterior subcapsular cataract looks like fine bubbles extending into the center of the pupil.

impeding vision. Vision becomes dimmer and blurrier, and you're likely to have trouble distinguishing colors. *Glare* might bother you, making it hard to drive at night. You may need stronger light for pursuits such as reading and needlework.

Cortical Cataracts

Many people develop *cortical cataracts* as they age. These cataracts begin as whitish, wedge-shaped opaque areas on the outer edge of the lens, near the capsular bag. Slowly, these opacities become streaks reaching inward to the center of the lens, like spokes on a wheel. When they reach the center, they block part of the light passing through the lens, and you will begin to have problems with blurry vision, especially in bright lights or nighttime glare. Cortical cataracts often require surgery at a comparatively early stage.

Subcapsular Cataracts

When a *subcapsular cataract* begins at the back of the lens, which is most often the case, it's called a *posterior subcapsular cataract*. It starts out as a grain-like opaque area on the capsular bag. Because posterior subcapsular cataracts are usually directly in the path of light on its way to the retina, you might have vision problems early, particularly driving into a setting sun.

Anyone can have subcapsular cataracts in one or both eyes. People who are extremely nearsighted, who have diabetes, or who have taken high doses of *steroids* are particularly at risk.

Can Cataracts Cause Blindness?

With continued neglect, a cataract may turn completely white. The pupil appears white instead of black. Described as *mature,* these cataracts are so advanced that the patient has little or no vision in the affected eye. Surgery is essential to remove the completely opaque lens before it becomes *hypermature.* In fact, it might be the white pupil that gave cataracts their name; the Latin term for "waterfall" is *cataracta.* The whitish color of a mature cataract is similar to the color of turbulent water, as in a waterfall. Surgery on a hypermature cataract is more difficult, and recovery takes longer than the usual lens replacement procedure. At one time, patients were advised to wait until their cataracts were mature, or "ripe," before having surgery. This approach was abandoned long ago. You would almost surely notice significant vision changes and seek treatment long before your cataracts were mature and visible to the naked eye.

Only if you ignore cataracts and fail to get proper treatment are they likely to cause blindness. There are a variety of reasons that cataracts go untreated. In some parts of the world, safe and effective cataract surgery is not readily available. Many people globally, unfortunately, do not have access to proper care or treatment, which is why cataracts are the most common cause of blindness worldwide. Even in the United States and other developed nations, however, many people are afraid to see a doctor about their failing vision. Some of them fear surgery, not realizing that lens replacement is a quick and virtually painless outpatient procedure with a very high success rate.

We've touched on signs and symptoms of cataracts. The next chapter will discuss these symptoms in greater detail and will help you and your doctor decide when it's time to consider surgery for your cataracts.

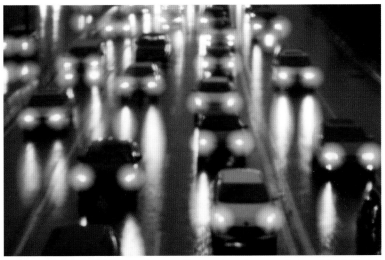

Cataracts cause overall blurring of vision. Glare, such as that seen during night driving, is also common.

Halos, Starbursts, and Glare

At night, your pupil gets bigger. A bigger pupil creates a larger pathway for light entering the eye, so more of the lens—including the edges of the cataract—is exposed. When bright light—car headlights, even street lighting and stoplights—enters the eye, the exposed cataract edges "scatter" the light, causing halos, starbursts, and glare. A *halo* is a circle of light around a light source. *Starbursts* are radiating lines of light coming out from the light. *Glare* is light that dazzles and seems almost blindingly bright. Glare most commonly happens when you're driving toward the setting sun.

You've experienced this scattering of light when you've driven at night with a fogged-up windshield. The tiny drops of moisture on the window bend the incoming light in multiple directions, in much the same way a cataract does, making it very difficult to see where you're going and unsafe to drive.

Loss of Contrast

Scattering of light inside the eye also causes *loss of contrast,* making it hard for you to distinguish the details of objects that are similar in tone to their surroundings. You might have trouble seeing a person's face when they are backlit against a window, or recognizing someone down a dimly lit hallway. Loss of contrast is scariest when it makes it hard to see the outline of a pedestrian in a crosswalk when you are driving at night or in bad weather.

Ghost Images and Double Vision

The tendency of cataracts to scatter light entering the lens can also cause ghost images or *double vision,* especially if you're looking at a light source, like a traffic light. With double vision, you'll see two relatively clear images, whereas *ghost images* are fainter "copies" that appear on one side of or around the object you are looking at.

Difficulty Seeing in Bright Light

In bright light the pupil becomes smaller, narrowing the pathway through which light enters the eye. A cataract located in the center of the lens can obstruct your vision more when your pupils are constricted. This happens most commonly when you are driving and turn toward the bright light of a setting sun. You can suddenly find yourself feeling blinded and needing to pull over.

Change in Color Vision

Age-related cataracts become grayish or yellowish as they thicken. Naturally, these tints affect your ability to distinguish colors. It's common for people with cataracts to report that blues and purples look washed-out and faded, and that whites appear yellowish. The world can look as if you are wearing dark yellow sunglasses.

Though cataracts are a normal consequence of aging, certain lifestyle, environmental, and health factors may cause cataracts to develop earlier for some people. We'll examine these factors in the next chapter.

4

What Causes Cataracts?

Most people get cataracts for no discernible reason. The cataracts are a normal part of aging. Asking what causes cataracts is like asking what causes gray hair or wrinkles—we don't know for sure. And, just like gray hair, everyone gets cataracts eventually, if they live long enough.

Why does this occur? The lens of the eye is made up mostly of water and protein. When we are young, the protein molecules within the lens are undamaged and allow us to see clearly. However, as we age, some of these molecules within the lens begin to break down and clouding develops. Smoking or obesity may accelerate this process. So, be kind to your body, to delay the onset of cataracts as long as possible.

Other Causes of Cataracts

In addition to aging, there are several other, less common, causes of cataracts.

Congenital Cataracts

In rare cases, babies are born with *congenital cataracts*. Mothers who get German measles (rubella) during the first three months of pregnancy are at high risk of having a baby with cataracts. Fortunately, now that people are routinely vaccinated

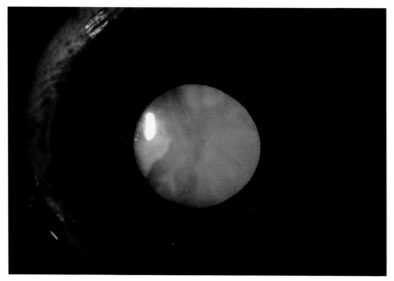

A severe cataract makes the lens completely white.

against rubella, this risk has virtually disappeared in the United States. Other infections and certain medications early in pregnancy can still cause congenital cataracts, as can hereditary conditions. These cataracts might or might not cause vision problems. If they do, they are surgically treated in much the same way as are cataracts in adults. Congenital cataracts are often quite small, and may not affect vision until middle age.

Illness-Related Cataracts

Diabetes mellitus is probably the most common source of cataracts that form due to disease. People with higher-than-normal blood sugar levels, even if they are not diabetic, are also at risk for cataracts. Certain eye diseases cause cataracts, particularly diseases that cause inflammation inside the eye. Some serious diseases require the long-term use of cortico-

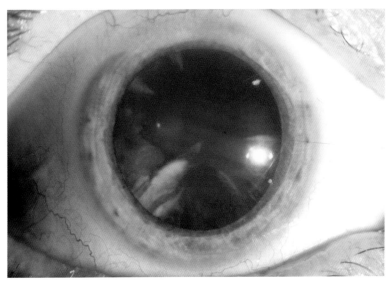

This is an example of mild cortical cataract. Vision is affected as the cataract reaches the center of the lens, causing glare and loss of contrast.

steroids, such as prednisone. These medications frequently cause cataracts after years of use, particularly if used as eye drops to treat eye inflammation.

Traumatic Cataracts

Eye injuries, caused by sharp objects or a direct blow to the eye, can cause *traumatic cataracts.* Traumatic cataracts may also form as a result of prior eye surgery. A blow to the head that misses the eye will not cause a cataract though.

Radiation

Radiation treatment to the head for cancer can cause cataracts. These usually develop years after the radiation treatment. There is some evidence that exposure to sunlight over many years can cause cataracts, too. Sunlight is most intense at the equator and may account for the higher incidence of cataracts among people who live near the equator.

Severe Nearsightedness

People who are severely nearsighted sometimes get cataracts in their fifties or sixties. We don't know why cataracts develop earlier in these people, but it may be related to degeneration of the protein gel that fills the eye.

Can You Prevent Cataracts?

You can't prevent cataracts entirely, but you might delay the onset of cataracts by being sensible about sun exposure, wearing UV-protective sunglasses when you're outdoors, eating well, and keeping fit. Delaying cataract formation may be just one of many benefits of a lifestyle that promotes health and well-being.

After your cataracts are diagnosed, it will be up to you to decide when they are unacceptably interfering with your work and your lifestyle. The next chapter contains guidelines for the timing of surgery.

5

When to Have Cataract Surgery

Cataract means that the lens in your eye has gotten hazy, so you are experiencing some of the symptoms we reviewed in chapter 3. Cataract surgery, simply put, is removing your old, hazy lens and replacing it with a new, clear, synthetic lens, called an *intraocular lens implant* or *IOL* for short.

Cataract surgery is painless and generally takes less than fifteen minutes. You are back to your work or usual activities the next day. Cataract surgery leads to better vision for nearly all patients—an astounding 98 percent, according to the Eye Surgery Education Council. This chapter reviews the issues you should consider in deciding when to have cataract surgery.

Clearing Up Misconceptions

First, let us clear up a few misconceptions. The first misconception is that there are treatments for cataracts other than surgery. There aren't. There are no eye drops that will reverse cataracts. There are no eye exercises that help. There are no vitamins or supplements that will clear up your vision. The only treatment for cataracts is cataract surgery.

The second misconception is that your cataracts have to be "ripe" before you can have surgery. That was a euphemism from the old days

(1970s) for saying that the cataract had to be quite advanced. That usually meant you had to be near blind before you could have surgery. At the time, cataract surgery techniques weren't very successful for mild cataracts. This is no longer the case. With modern techniques, cataract surgeons can treat even minimal cataracts safely.

That doesn't mean, though, that everyone with cataracts should have cataract surgery. Cataract surgery, while very safe, still has some risks (these are reviewed in detail in chapter 8). The decision to have cataract surgery, like any surgery, requires us to balance the benefits of surgery against these uncommon risks. When you first develop a cataract, surgery is usually not the initial step in managing the problem. In a cataract's early stages, getting stronger glasses or contacts often is all you need to see clearly. Using a magnifying glass, a page magnifier, or better lighting can help. Patients with early cataracts may find that their vision is fine for most activities except night driving. Perhaps your spouse can do more of the driving at night.

In general, if you can function well in your daily life with glasses, we recommend you delay surgery. On the other hand, if you find that your optimal functioning is impaired in important ways, and glasses don't solve the problem, then we recommend proceeding with surgery.

Are Your Cataracts Bad Enough for Surgery?

In addition to death and taxes, the other certainty in life is that cataracts always get worse over time. Eventually your cataracts will become more than an inconvenience. At some point stronger glasses or contacts, magnifying devices, better lighting, and other interim measures won't be sufficient to keep you seeing the way you want to see. Then it is time to have cataract surgery. Here are some of the factors that might help you make your decision:

- *You feel unsafe driving.* Glare when you are driving into the setting sun may seem blinding to you. It is hard to read street signs, so you are uncomfortable driving out of your usual neighborhood. There is glare around lights, particularly oncoming headlights, that makes it hard to drive at night.

- *You feel a loss of independence.* You may have trouble seeing curbs or steps or irregularities in the pavement, so you are afraid of stumbling or falling. One study looked at Medicare patients who had cataract surgery, and found they had a lower risk of hip fracture, presumably because they could walk more confidently.

- *Your vision isn't good enough for you to work accurately.* This can be particularly a problem working with numbers or spreadsheets, where it is easy to confuse a 3 with an 8 or a 6. If you do lots of reading, you may find that your poor vision is slowing down your ability to work efficiently.

- *Vision problems due to cataracts are diminishing your quality of life.* If you're an avid reader, photographer, cyclist, or golfer, for example, your cataracts might make these pursuits more difficult or less enjoyable than they could be.

Life is short, and we want our time on Earth to be as fulfilling as possible. If your quality of life is limited by these issues, it's probably time for surgery.

Limitations of Cataract Surgery

Almost anyone who has cataracts and who is in reasonably good health, regardless of age, can have cataract surgery. There are a few things to keep in mind, however.

Remember that cataract surgery corrects only cataracts and won't fix other eye problems. For example, people with macular degeneration who have cataracts may have some vision loss from the cataract and some vision loss from the macular degeneration. Fixing the cataract will make the vision better, but it will still be limited somewhat by the macular degeneration. If you have other eye diseases, ask your doctor how well you can expect to see after cataract surgery.

Sometimes coexisting eye diseases can be treated at the same time as the cataract. Glaucoma is an example. Glaucoma is a disease caused by too much pressure in the eye. During cataract surgery, the surgeon may be able to place a microscopic shunt that relieves the pressure in your eye, treating both the cataract and the glaucoma at the same session.

The goal of modern cataract surgery is to give you excellent vision without glasses for many of your activities. This is liberating for many, and especially wonderful for extremely nearsighted or farsighted people who have had to wear thick glasses their entire life. However, we don't always achieve excellent vision without glasses, so you may need to wear glasses most of the time after surgery. If you have had previous vision correction surgery, like LASIK, the calculation of lens implant power is somewhat more complicated and somewhat less precise.

Don't expect the impossible. Modern cataract surgery can free you from glasses much of the time, but usually not all of the time. Most people still wear glasses sometimes, often for reading. In all likelihood, you'll be delighted with the improvement in your eyesight—as long as you don't expect to see as well as you did in your twenties.

Is It Risky to Delay Cataract Surgery?

The short answer to this question is no. There is never a need to rush into cataract surgery. Cataracts are not like cancer—there is not a danger in delaying treatment. If you are unsure about whether it is time to proceed, it is fine to wait. Surgery can always be done later.

On the other hand, some people wait until the cataracts are well advanced. They might fear surgery, or believe that poor eyesight is just "part of getting older." This makes us sad. We as surgeons know that they have missed important parts of life as their vision got worse. Their life would have been richer and more enjoyable had they not waited so long. The fact is, the many benefits of cataract removal and lens replacement greatly outweigh the slight risks.

New techniques make the cataract surgery procedure quick and painless; you can have surgery first thing in the morning and be home in time for lunch. Within a day you can be back at work, already enjoying your clear vision and your independence.

You might have a newfound freedom from glasses and contacts. The next chapter explains how modern cataract surgery achieves these miracles.

Modern Cataract Surgery: An Overview

Because virtually everyone eventually develops cataracts, and because cataract surgery is so safe and effective, it is the most commonly done surgical procedure in the United States. The procedure takes less than fifteen minutes. Recovery is so rapid that most people notice dramatic improvements in vision by the next morning. This chapter reviews the advances that make modern cataract surgery possible.

Removing the Old Lens

Cataract surgery involves removing your old lens and inserting a new lens implant to give you clear vision. Although cataract surgery is very common and highly successful, the procedure itself is more challenging than it may sound. To give you the fast recovery that is a hallmark of modern cataract surgery, we use very small incisions, only 2.5 mm wide. That is less than one-eighth of an inch wide. These incisions are so small that no sutures are needed—the incisions seal themselves.

The challenging part is this: your cloudy natural lens is a fat disk, 12 mm across and 4 mm thick. To remove this through a 2.5 mm incision is like trying to fit a camel through the eye of a needle! We solve this problem by breaking the cataract into small pieces, either by cracking it with instruments or by using a laser. Then the pieces are vacuumed from the eye with a tiny ultrasonic probe.

Inserting a New Lens

After the cataract is out of the eye, the new lens implant needs to be inserted. Here the same problem occurs again: the new lens is 6 mm wide (1/4 inch) wide and 12 mm (just under 1/2 inch) long, and it needs to fit through a 2.5 mm incision. We solve this problem by folding up the new lens implant up into a tight roll, and injecting it into the eye through

Manual Cataract Surgery

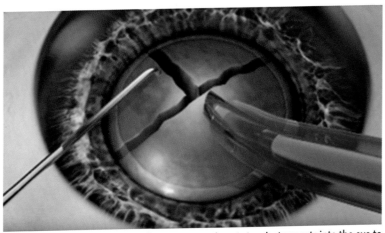

During manual cataract surgery, the eye surgeon inserts two instruments into the eye to crack the cataract into tiny pieces, that are then removed.

a 2.4 mm tube that just fits inside the incision. The lens is unrolled in the eye and positioned in place of the old lens.

It gets even more challenging. As described in chapter 1, the lens is built like a peach, in three layers. There is an inner core, called the *nucleus,* corresponding to the pit of the peach. There is a thin outer layer, called the *capsular bag,* which corresponds to the skin of the peach. Finally there is a layer between the capsular bag and the nucleus, called the *cortex,* corresponding to the flesh of the peach.

The surgeon's goal is to remove the inner two layers, the nucleus and cortex, and leave the thin outer layer, the capsular bag. It is very important to leave the capsular bag because the new lens implant is placed inside it; the capsular bag surrounds the new lens implant and holds it in place. This can be challenging. The capsular bag is about as thin as a piece of tissue paper and almost as fragile. Cataract surgery can damage the capsular bag. If the capsular bag is damaged, it may not be possible to insert the chosen lens implant, or any implant at all. Laser cataract surgery, discussed later, offers in our opinion a safer approach to cataract surgery that lessens the risk of damage to the capsular bag.

If the description of cataract surgery in the prior paragraphs sounds complicated to you, you are right. And it is even more complicated than that. In the next sections, we take you step by step through a modern cataract procedure. First we describe traditional manual cataract surgery, then we explain how that differs from the more modern laser cataract surgery.

Manual Cataract Surgery

Manual cataract surgery is the traditional procedure, and is still the way the majority of cataract surgeries are performed (although not in our practice). Manual surgery involves inserting instruments into the eye and using them to crack the cataract into pieces that are small enough to be removed from the eye. In this section we describe the process of undergoing manual cataract surgery. In the next section we'll describe how laser cataract surgery differs.

Having surgery on your eyes may sound scary. We want you to be calm and relaxed, so before the surgery starts you will be sedated. In the operating room, intravenous anesthesia is given by the anesthesiologist. This is usually a combination of a sedative and a pain reliever to ensure your comfort. The sedation is very similar to that used for colonoscopy.

The goal is not to put you to sleep but rather to make you so relaxed and drowsy that you don't care that someone is operating on your eye. Patients often do fall asleep anyway. Regardless of whether or not you fall asleep, we make sure you are calm, comfortable, and relaxed. Numbing eye drops are given to give you an extra layer of protection against pain. At that point the surgery begins.

Step 1: Preparation. After you are relaxed and comfortable, the surgeon makes two small incisions at the *limbus* (the junction between the white and colored part of your eye). The larger incision is a tiny 2.5 mm wide, and the smaller incision is only 1 mm wide. The two incisions allow the surgeon to use two instruments in your eye, one in each hand. The surgeon then injects numbing medicine directly inside the eye. Next her or she injects a jellylike substance that replaces the fluid in the front of the eye. This helps the eye hold its shape as the cataract is removed.

Step 2: Perform the capsulorhexis. We described the capsular bag previously, and its importance to the surgery. The surgeon needs to get to the nucleus and cortex to remove them, but the capsular bag is in the way, so the surgeon needs to remove the front part of the capsular bag. The surgeon does this by tearing the front of the capsular bag in a carefully controlled fashion to create a 5-mm hole in the capsular bag. This tear is called the *capsulorhexis.* It is a particularly tricky part of the surgery when done manually. (It is much easier to do with the laser, as described later.) Just beneath this hole lie the cortex and nucleus, ready for removal.

Laser Cataract Surgery

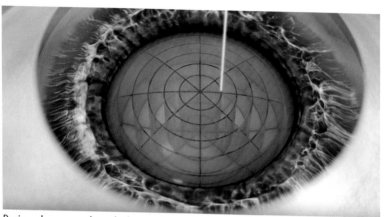

During a laser procedure, the laser softens and breaks up the cataract. Then the pieces are easily removed.

Step 3: Break up the nucleus. The nucleus is usually hard, like the pit in the peach analogy above. In traditional surgery, the nucleus is broken up by hand. The surgeon holds one instrument in each hand, and compresses the nucleus between the two instruments. This pressure cracks the nucleus in half. The surgeon then rotates the nucleus and repeats this process a number of times, gradually shattering the nucleus into small pieces. This is a tricky part of the surgery because the instruments can damage the capsular bag. (In laser cataract surgery, this step is done automatically by the laser; *see* below.)

Step 4. Vacuum out the pieces of nucleus. The nucleus now consists of a number of small fragments, but each of these pieces is still hard. The surgeon removes these pieces using a small handheld ultrasonic probe. The probe's microscopic high-speed vibration breaks up (emulsifies) the small pieces and vacuums them out of your eye. This process is called *phacoemulsification.*

Step 5. Clean up the cortex. After the nucleus is removed, there is still the lens cortex left. The cortex is the flesh of the peach in the analogy above. The cortex is removed by vacuuming it out of the eye, just like the nucleus fragments. Then the surgeon polishes the capsular bag so it is clean and clear, ready to accept the new lens implant.

Step 6. Implant the new lens. The new lens implant is rolled up by the surgical technician and inserted into a short tube, called a *cartridge*. The surgeon inserts the cartridge into the incision and activates a plunger to push the new lens implant through the cartridge into the eye. Once in the eye, the new lens implant unfurls by itself. The surgeon gently pushes the implant through the opening in the front of the capsular bag, and seats the implant inside the capsular bag. The lens implant has two protrusions, called *haptics,* sticking out from each edge. These haptics push on the "equator" of the capsular bag and keep the lens implant centered and stable forever. Manual cataract surgery is a sophisticated operation and is remarkably successful at restoring vision lost to cataracts.

In the next section we describe a new level of refinement of cataract surgery: laser cataract surgery.

Laser Cataract Surgery

First, a bit of surgical philosophy: the best way to make a surgical procedure safer is to make the hardest parts of the surgery easier. Use of the laser in cataract surgery does exactly that. In particular, the laser creates the capsulorhexis effortlessly and the laser breaks up the nucleus, so it does not have to be broken up manually.

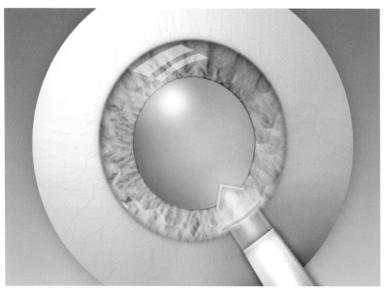

During cataract surgery, a small incision is made in the cornea.

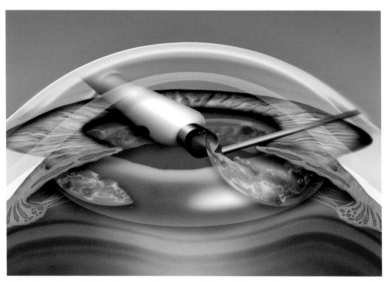

After the cataract is broken up, either manually or by laser, the surgeon vacuums the pieces of cataract out of the eye with an ultrasonic suction probe.

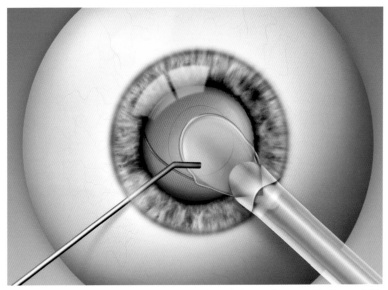

The new lens implant is rolled up and inserted through the small incision. The lens unfolds itself.

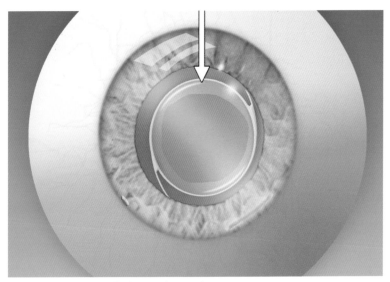

The eye with the intraocular lens implant in place.

The laser that is used is called the *femtosecond laser.* This laser is able to create precise cuts in the eye by connecting together hundreds of thousands of tiny laser pulses. It was originally introduced in 2001 for performing LASIK surgery to correct nearsightedness. It wasn't long before some cataract experts realized it could make cataract surgery significantly easier.

Laser cataract surgery goes by several names. Some people call it *femtosecond laser cataract surgery.* Some call it by the acronym *FLACS,* which stands for *femtosecond laser-assisted cataract surgery.* We prefer the simpler *laser cataract surgery.*

Regardless of the name used, a laser cataract surgery procedure starts with using the laser to break up the cataract, even before the first incision is made. The patient is taken to the laser room and given sedation. The eye is numbed using eye drops. The eye is measured using a scanning laser, which outlines the exact dimensions of the cataract and the location of the various eye structures like the iris and the capsular bag that must be avoided during laser treatment.

The femtosecond laser is then activated to create a perfect circular opening (capsulorhexis) in the front of the capsular bag. The laser then cuts the lens nucleus into small pieces. If astigmatism correction is desired, the laser then creates tiny arc-like incisions near the edge of the cornea to correct the astigmatism. We use the laser to make these incisions routinely in patients with a low level of astigmatism, as we try to perfect the vision after surgery. Higher degrees of astigmatism can be treated with incisions, too, but are generally more accurately treated with a *toric lens* implant instead, as described later in this chapter.

Single Focus Intraocular Lens

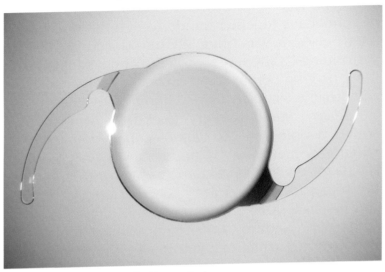

A traditional single focus, standard intraocular lens.

Laser Procedure Is Painless

The entire measurement and laser treatment process is painless and takes less than two minutes. At the completion of the laser treatment, the surgeon then performs the remainder of the cataract surgery. The rest of the surgery is similar to manual cataract surgery, with important differences. Rather than repeat each of the steps in manual surgery, described above, we just highlight the differences below. Similar to manual surgery, you will be very sedated and comfortable before the procedure starts.

Step 1: Preparation. This step is the same.

Step 2: Perform the capsulorhexis. In manual cataract surgery, the surgeon tears an opening in the capsule of the lens. Sometimes the capsular bag has a mind of its own and tears in the wrong direction. Sometimes the hole is too small, and it is difficult to get the pieces of nucleus out through the hole. Sometimes the hole is too big, and the edge of the lens implant pops in front of the capsular bag after surgery. Sometimes the hole is off-center, so the lens doesn't center properly.

With the laser, there is no need for the surgeon to tear an opening in the capsular bag by hand. The opening has already been made by the laser, with exceptional precision. The laser is designed to create a perfectly round opening that is well centered and has just the right diameter. This helps ensure your lens implant stays exactly in the optimal position for the rest of your life.

Step 3: Break up the nucleus. Breaking up the nucleus is the other most challenging part of cataract surgery. In manual surgery, the surgeon needs to fracture the lens by squeezing it between two instruments. The force applied can sometimes drive one of these instruments, the phacoemulsification needle, through the back part of the capsular bag. That is a potentially serious complication of cataract surgery. (*See* chapter 8 for more details.)

In laser cataract surgery, the laser cuts the nucleus into small pieces before the procedure starts. There is no need for the surgeon to crack the nucleus into pieces. One carefully controlled, randomized study found the rate of damage to the back part of the capsular bag was 3 percent with manual surgery and 0 percent with laser cataract surgery.

Step 4. Vacuum out the pieces of nucleus. This step is identical to Step 4 of manual cataract surgery. The surgeon removes the small pieces of cataract created in the previous step using a small handheld ultrasonic probe.

Step 5. Clean up the cortex. This step is identical to Step 5 of manual cataract surgery. After the nucleus is removed, there is still lens cortex left. The cortex is removed by vacuuming it out of the eye, just like the nucleus fragments.

Step 6. Implant the new lens. This step is also the same as Step 6 of manual surgery. The new lens implant is rolled up and inserted into the eye. The surgeon gently seats the implant inside the capsular bag.

Lens Implants

Cataract surgery removes your natural lens because it has become cloudy. A replacement is necessary. A key component of modern cataract surgery is the choice of the best lens implant for your eye. You likely will be qualified for a number of options, and, with the help of your doctor, you will need to pick one. No matter which implant you choose, the new lens becomes part of the eye. It is safe, stable, and reliable, it requires no care or maintenance, and it lasts forever. This section gives you the information you need to help you pick the best lens implant for your eye.

Think of your range of vision as encompassing three zones: far vision, intermediate vision, and near vision. Far vision is the zone from about 5 feet away out to infinity. Intermediate vision is the zone at arm's length, the range of a computer or the dashboard on your car. Near vision is the zone about 14 to 20 inches away. Near vision is the zone you are using when you read a book or a newspaper or a mobile phone.

Multifocal Lens Implant

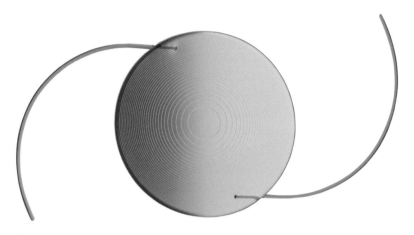

This multifocal lens implant provides a wide range of vision, both near and distant. The "bullseye" rings in the lens make this possible.

Monovision Implants:
One Eye for Distance and One Eye for Reading

Normally, an eye can only see at one of the three zones listed above. Since we have two eyes, an option to provide a greater range of vision is to correct one eye for the distance zone and one eye for the reading zone. This arrangement is called *monovision.* Monovision is confusing name. It should be called bivision because the eyes cover two different distances. Unfortunately, we are stuck with the name.

Some people as they age wear contact lenses that create monovision, with one eye for distance and one eye for reading. These lucky people don't have to wear reading glasses. Surgeons can create the same condition by using lens implants of different powers in the two eyes. In that way, patients can see far and near without glasses.

Monovision is not for everyone. Monovision will cover the distance and close zones, but patients with monovision generally still need glasses for computer use, and other things in the intermediate zone of vision. Also, monovision involves creating an intentional imbalance between the eyes. Sometimes with monovision the eyes don't work well together. In this case you would have to wear glasses to make the eyes work together, which defeats the purpose of the monovision. For this reason, surgeons generally don't recommend monovision unless the patient has tolerated monovision contacts in the past. We discuss monovision here because it is an option with many of our lens implants to extend the range of vision in selected patients.

Standard Lens Implants

Lens implants fall into two general categories: standard lens implants and advanced lens implants. Standard lens implants are designed to work with glasses to give you good vision. These lenses may give good vision in a single zone—distance, intermediate, or near—without glasses, or they may not (depending on your astigmatism). For the other two zones, you will definitely need glasses. In contrast, advanced lens implants are designed to give good vision without glasses, and often good vision without glasses in two or all three of the zones described above.

The first decision you need to make is: do you mind wearing glasses much or all of the time? If the answer is that you don't mind wearing glasses much of the time, a standard lens implant is probably the right choice for you. Standard lens implants work well for two types of people. First, if you don't mind wearing glasses all the time, standard lens implants

Light-Adjustable Lens

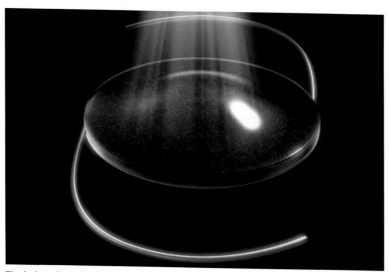

The light-adjustable lens is made of silicone that can be shaped by ultraviolet light after the lens is placed in the eye. This process allows for the correction of any remaining nearsightedness, farsightedness, and astigmatism after cataract surgery.

are great. Second, if you have low astigmatism and want to see at a single range (distance, intermediate, or near) without glasses, a standard lens can give you good vision without glasses at that particular range. That is because a standard implant is a *monofocal lens* implant; that is, it has a single point of focus. This implant is similar to the lens in a disposable camera—it can't change its focus. Usually these lenses provide good mid-distance vision, and you will wear glasses for all other distances. If you have previously tolerated monovision (discussed above) with contact lenses, then standard lens implants can also be used to create monovision.

Advanced Lens Implants

Nobody has cataract surgery for fun—it is innately scary and a big decision for many people. We find that most people feel that, if they must go through it, they might as well have the best lens implant possible. If you want a higher degree of freedom from glasses, or an increased range of vision without glasses, then an advanced lens implant is probably the right choice.

Advanced lens implants use a range of technologies to reduce your dependency on eyeglasses after cataract surgery. The various advanced lens implants are discussed in this section. Each type has its own unique set of advantages.

Toric Lens Implant

If you have significant astigmatism, the *toric lens* implant is a great option. It is designed to correct your astigmatism, thereby providing sharper vision with less reliance on glasses. If astigmatism is not corrected, it affects all types of vision, including near vision, intermediate vision, and distance vision. Glasses would be required for most activities. The toric lens implant doesn't give an increased range of vision, but it does give excellent vision in the zone of your choice: either distance or intermediate or near. If toric lenses are implanted in both eyes for distance vision, then reading glasses would need to be used for intermediate and near vision. Alternatively, the toric lens can be used to create monovision, with one eye corrected for distance while the other eye is corrected for near vision, thereby reducing the need for reading glasses. Mild levels of astigmatism do not require a toric lens implant, because the other advanced lens implants can correct mild astigmatism in addition to their other benefits, which are described below.

Accommodating Lens Implant

An *accommodating lens* implant is designed like a normal, young human lens, where the focusing muscle of the eye is able to alter the position or shape of the lens, leading to improved ability to focus. As we write, the only accommodating lens available is the *Crystalens*. However, the Crystalens is not often used because it doesn't give much near vision, and distance vision can decline over a period of years as the lens compresses with natural healing. We prefer the light-adjustable lens (*see* section below) for patients who want excellent distance vision or monovision, because it is much more precise than any other lens.

Multifocal Lens Implant

This lens is called multifocal because it has two focal points. It corrects for both distance vision and near vision simultaneously. A *multifocal lens* implant usually allows you to read and see far away without glasses. This implant offers the greatest freedom from glasses. It does, however, have two significant limitations.

First, this implant causes rings around lights at night, called *halos*. Halos are usually not bothersome but can be annoying during night driving. Second, this implant sacrifices some clarity of distance vision, which may be especially noticeable at night, in dim light, or in fog. Most patients like the multifocal lens because of the increased range of vision, but those who are unhappy are generally unhappy because they feel like there is a film over their distance vision. If you do a lot of driving at night, or perform delicate, detailed, close work, another implant is probably a better choice for you. Also, as with all implants, you shouldn't expect perfection: reading glasses may be needed at times for small print.

Extended-Range Implant

The *extended-range lens* implant falls in between the standard lens implant and multifocal lens implants. The extended-range lens offers very crisp distance vision—better than multifocal lenses. It also offers very good intermediate vision—better than the standard lens implants. You may hear it referred to as an *extended-depth-of-focus (EDOF)* lens. This lens allows you to read your cell phone or a menu at arm's length. On the other hand, it usually does not allow you to read a book or newspaper without glasses. It also causes some halos around lights at night, although these are usually not bothersome. The extended-range lens is best for patients who want excellent, crisp distance vision and the ability to read at arm's length without glasses.

Light-Adjustable Lens Implant

Cataract surgeons do a careful and detailed calculation of the lens implant power you need to get excellent vision without glasses. These calculations are quite good, but nowhere near 100 percent accurate. Also, each person heals a little differently, so even a perfect calculation is partially undone by normal healing. Today, despite the slight inaccuracies, most people get very good vision without glasses, but often not perfect vision. Even with the best preoperative measurements and calculations, slightly less than half of patients get perfect 20/20 vision.

The *light-adjustable* lens is a remarkable lens implant whose power can be adjusted after surgery by shining an ultraviolet light on the lens. By precisely controlling the pattern of light, the lens implant power can be adjusted to correct any remaining myopia, hyperopia, or astigmatism. The result is extraordinarily clear 20/20 vision in the great majority of patients. There is no need to undergo an additional surgical procedure like LASIK for perfect vision.

The light-adjustable lens does require a greater commitment from you. Because ultraviolet light changes the lens power, you need to wear sunglasses outdoors for the first few weeks after surgery. It also requires extra visits to the doctor, because the adjustment of the lens power is done in one or two steps, followed by a lock-in step that freezes the power of the lens permanently, so it is no longer affected by sunlight. We see it as a twenty-second-century technology that arrived a century early!

Switching Lens Implants

If you've read the prior section carefully, you may feel that the choice of the correct implant is tricky. The good news is this: it is usually an easy decision. The surgeon and his or her staff will guide you to the right decision.

You may wonder, what if I pick the wrong implant? Fortunately, that is only a minor problem. If the implant isn't right for you, for whatever reason, it is generally easy to go back to the operating room and switch it out for a different implant. Obviously, no one wants to do another surgery, but the important message is that you aren't stuck for the rest of your life with a lens implant that you are unhappy with.

Enhancement Surgery

Our goal with advanced implants is to give you excellent vision without glasses. To help us achieve this, each of the implants described above comes in a large range of powers. Before surgery we measure your eye carefully and calculate the exact lens power needed to give you the best vision (these measurements are described in the next chapter).

Unfortunately, the calculations are not perfectly precise, and each person's healing is slightly different. This means that, despite our best efforts, your eye may turn out to have a little nearsightedness or farsightedness or astigmatism after surgery. That means that, despite the advanced implant you have in your eye, you may still have to wear glasses to get great vision. Needless to say, that can be disappointing.

Don't worry! If you do have nearsightedness or farsightedness or astigmatism after surgery, it can be corrected with a LASIK procedure. You have probably heard about *LASIK*—it is a popular in-office laser procedure that helps eliminate the need to wear glasses. It works equally well in people who have had cataract surgery. If your vision is not good enough after the cataract surgery, a LASIK procedure can usually be done to sharpen it up. Another advantage of the light-adjustable implant is that enhancement is almost never needed.

We have tried to give you a perspective in this chapter on the remarkable sophistication and variety that characterize modern cataract surgery. If the procedure sounds hopelessly complicated to you, rest assured that, in expert hands, the procedure is elegant, quick, and highly successful.

Now that you have had a high-level view of the procedure, we take you in the next chapter through the practicalities of the cataract eye examination.

6

The Preoperative Eye Examination

Eye surgery is one of the most advanced fields of medicine. Eye doctors use amazingly sophisticated machines to examine your eyes, machines that can see a single cell inside your eye. In this chapter, we review the preoperative visit, where your cataract is diagnosed and the surgery is planned. The preoperative eye examination gives you and your doctor information about the overall health of your eyes and about other conditions that might be affecting your eyesight. The exam reveals how much of your vision loss is due to cataracts rather than other eye diseases, like macular degeneration or glaucoma.

Different Types of Eye Doctor

In the United States, comprehensive eye exams can be performed by ophthalmologists and optometrists. Both are eye doctors, but their training and practice are different.

An *ophthalmologist* is a medical doctor (M.D.), like an orthopedic surgeon, neurosurgeon, or plastic surgeon, who has completed medical school, an internship, and an ophthalmology residency to learn the medicine and surgery of the eyes, eyelids, and ocular system. Cataract surgery is done by an

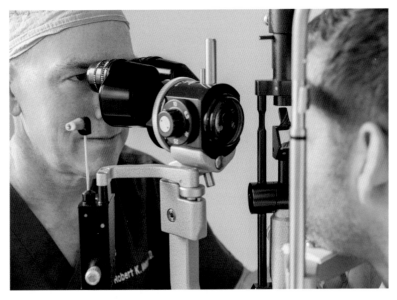

Dr. Maloney is shown using a slit lamp to perform a microscopic evaluation of the interior of the eyes and to assess the degree of cataract formation.

ophthalmologist. Cataract and refractive surgeons are ophthalmologists who further specialize in surgical correction of vision and focusing problems.

An *optometrist,* or doctor of optometry (O.D.), specializes in primary eye care, including vision correction and medical conditions of the eye. Optometrists can prescribe glasses, contact lenses, and medications, but they do not perform surgery. If an optometrist diagnoses cataracts or eye disease, he or she will refer the patient to an ophthalmologist for surgical treatment, when necessary. Many optometrists work closely with ophthalmologists in the preoperative and postoperative care of cataract surgery patients. Commonly, the ophthalmologist surgeon performs the cataract surgery and the optometrist does the postoperative care.

How Do I Find a Cataract Surgeon?

The best source of referrals is other eye specialists. Ask your optometrist or primary care physician to recommend a surgeon. Look for a surgeon who does a lot of surgery, because practice makes perfect. Many ophthalmologists do general eye care as well as cataract surgery. These surgeons often have significantly less experience, because they are busy doing lots of things other than cataract surgery. Make sure to pick a surgeon who uses advanced lenses and does laser cataract surgery. You should be able to find this information on the surgeon's website.

Another good source of referrals is "best-of" lists. "Best Doctors in America" and "America's Best Doctors" compile a list every year of doctors recommended by other expert physicians. Check out the surgeon's reviews online. These reviews will give you an idea of how satisfied his or her patients are. Ask people who have had cataract surgery what they think of their surgeon. Other patients can tell you how the doctor and the doctor's office treated them.

Preparing for Your Eye Exam

Before you go to your appointment, assemble your medical records. Your eye doctor will want information about:

- any past eye disorders, injuries, and operations
- your contact lens prescription for each eye, if you wear contacts
- past and present medical problems
- all medications you're taking, including contraceptives and other prescription drugs

- over-the-counter medications, herbs, and homeopathic products, as well as food supplements such as vitamins and minerals
- any family history of eye disease
- your occupation and hobbies (in order to determine the potential for injury and also to understand how you use your eyes—primarily for driving or computer work, for example)
- the name, address, and phone number of your regular eye doctor and your primary care physician.

Be sure to take your eyeglasses or contact lenses to your appointment. Take sunglasses, too, because your doctor will probably use eye drops to dilate your pupils, which will make your eyes sensitive to bright light for several hours. In fact, you might want to arrange for someone to drive you home.

Comprehensive Eye Examination

In a routine comprehensive exam, the doctor will check your eyes for a variety of conditions, including:

- *refractive error* (whether or not glasses will help your vision)
- *strabismus* ("cross-eye") and *amblyopia* ("lazy eye")
- *glaucoma* (high pressure within the eye)
- *cataracts* (clouding of the natural lens)
- *macular degeneration* (deterioration of the macula)
- other, rarer eye diseases

Visual Acuity Test

The term *visual acuity* refers to the clarity of your vision. (*Acuity* is from the Latin *acuitas,* which means

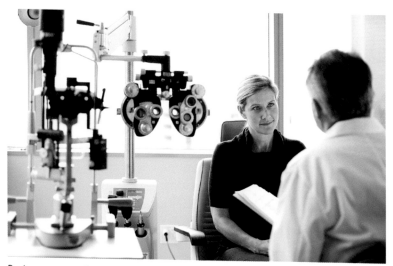

During your appointment, your eye doctor will want information about any past eye disorders and your medical history.

"sharpness.") In other words, how well do you see? Your eye doctor will probably use the familiar eye chart to test your vision at various distances. The eye chart most of us know is called the *Snellen chart,* after the nineteenth-century Dutch ophthalmologist Hermann Snellen, who invented it. It consists of rows of black letters—very large at the top, very small at the bottom—against a white background. Each eye will be tested separately while the other eye is covered.

The results of your visual acuity test are expressed by phrases such as "20/20 vision" and "20/40 vision," which some people find confusing. The first number in the phrase, in the United States at least, is always 20—which is the distance, in feet, you're standing from the eye chart. (Where the metric system is used, the first number is 6, indicating that the patient is standing 6 meters from the chart.)

The second number conveys how much your visual acuity differs from "normal" eyesight. If you have *20/20 vision,* you can see at 20 feet what other people with good vision can see at 20 feet. If your vision is 20/40, you can see at 20 feet what people with good vision can see at 40 feet. The higher the second number, the worse your visual acuity. At 20/200—meaning that someone with "normal" vision standing 200 feet away can see the chart as well as you can at 20 feet away—you are considered legally blind. (Only about 10 percent of *legally blind* Americans have zero visual acuity; the rest have some degree of sight.)

Refractive Error Testing

The doctor will perform a test to determine your degree of farsightedness, nearsightedness, or astigmatism. This is called your refractive error. The doctor will also determine how well you can see with an optimal eyeglass prescription. This is important; if glasses correct your vision well, you don't need cataract surgery. Instead you need a new pair of eyeglasses.

To measure refractive error precisely, the doctor will use a device called a *phoropter.* If you've had an eye exam, you're probably familiar with a phoropter. It is a complete range of corrective lenses that can be adjusted to offer you hundreds of combinations. The doctor adjusts the lenses and asks you, "Which is better, one or two?" By continually changing the lenses, the doctor can arrive at a combination of lens strengths that will optimize your vision.

Eye Movement Testing

The doctor tests for crossed eyes by asking you to look upward and downward, and to the right and the left. You may be asked to stare at an object—first at a distance and later up close. The doctor may cover one of your eyes and quickly note how much the uncovered eye moves to adjust.

Visual Field Testing

The simplest way to test your *field of vision*—how far you can see to the left and right out of the corners of your eyes—is for you to focus on the doctor's face while he or she holds up fingers off to the side and asks you to report how many fingers you can see. Devices such as the *perimeter,* which emits flashes of light in the periphery eliciting patient response, are used to reveal visual field defects (abnormal blind spots).

Eye Pressure Measurement

Your eye doctor will probably use a tonometer to screen your eyes for glaucoma. Some tonometers expel a puff of air toward the eye and measure the resulting small, instantaneous indentation. The size of the indentation indicates the *intraocular pressure* inside the eye. Other types of tonometers are placed directly on the cornea to measure pressure, after the eye is numbed with eye drops.

Slit Lamp Examination

A *slit lamp,* or *biomicroscope,* is an examining microscope that allows the doctor to examine the structures of your eye closely. During a slit lamp exam, your head will be comfortably stabilized on the lamp's chin rest and the doctor evaluates the eyes for signs of disease at the front of the eye, including problems in the eyelids, tear film, cornea, *conjunctiva,* and iris. Using a higher-powered lens, he or she can also see to the back of the eye, detecting macular degeneration and other retinal problems.

As its name suggests, the slit lamp shines a slit of light into the eye. The size of the slit is adjustable, so the doctor can see very small sections of the eye at very high magnification. The slit lamp allows a clear view of the lens of the eye, and is the primary method by which cataracts are diagnosed.

Dilating the Pupils

For certain additional tests—to examine your general eye health and the retina, optic nerve, and blood vessels—the doctor will often need to dilate your pupils using eye drops. These drops take about thirty minutes to fully open the pupils, giving the doctor a much wider view of the inside of your eyes than would be possible with constricted pupils.

After dilation of your pupils, your vision might be blurred and highly sensitive to light for several hours. You won't want to walk out into bright sunlight with your eyes uncovered. If you don't have sunglasses, most eye doctors will give you disposable sunglasses to wear on the way home. Since there's no way of knowing how long it will take your eyes to return to normal, the best course is to arrange for someone to drive you home.

Ophthalmoscopic Examination

An *ophthalmoscope* is a specialized device through which your doctor can inspect the blood vessels and the optic nerve at the back of the eye. He or she will also examine the retina for detachment and tears, and the small area on the retina responsible for sharpest vision, the macula.

Potential Acuity Testing

If you have cataracts, the doctor may perform *potential acuity testing,* an estimate of what your vision would be like if the cataracts were removed. Potential acuity testing is especially useful in determining how much of your vision loss is due to cataracts. One way of testing potential acuity is with a retinal acuity meter, which projects an eye chart directly onto the retina, bypassing the cataract. You are asked to read it out loud, just like the chart on the wall.

Calculating the Power of Your News Lens Implant

Each lens implant is made in a variety of different powers. It is important to pick the right power implant to optimize your vision after the surgery. A very important part of the cataract preoperative exam is measuring your eye to calculate the lens implant power. This process is called *biometry.* A scanning laser is used to measure the dimensions of your eye—its length, corneal curvature, corneal diameter, and lens thickness. The surgeon uses these measurements to calculate the lens implant power.

If you are having an advanced lens implant, the surgeon should also do *corneal topography.* Corneal topography uses reflected light to create a precise three-dimensional map of the cornea, much like the topographic map of a mountain range. This allows more accurate correction of your astigmatism during the surgery.

Contact lenses can slightly distort the shape of your eye, which affects biometry. For the most accurate measurements, keep soft contact lenses out of your eyes for three days before your evaluation. If you wear hard contacts or rigid gas permeable (RGP) contacts, stop wearing them two weeks before the evaluation. Discontinuing contact lenses allows your eyes to return to their normal shape.

Education

A very important part of the comprehensive examination is educating you about the cataract surgery as it applies to your eye. This includes helping you pick the right lens implant and provides useful general information about the surgery, but your eye exam will provide information that is particular to *your* eyes. At the end of the preoperative examination, you should understand what's wrong with your eyes and how the doctor plans to fix it. At that point you are ready to schedule your cataract procedure.

7

Your Cataract Procedure

In this chapter, we will give you an idea of what it is like to go through cataract surgery, how to prepare for the procedure, and what to expect afterward. The process we describe here is what we do in our center, but it applies quite well no matter where you have surgery. If your surgeon gives you instructions different from those here, obviously follow his or her instructions rather than ours.

Countdown to Surgery

You've already had your preoperative consultation, described in the prior chapter. You've chosen a lens implant and signed all the required forms. You've scheduled your surgery. There are still a few things to be done leading up to the day of the procedure.

A Few Weeks before Surgery

You will receive twilight sedation at the time of your surgery with medicines through an IV line. Intravenous sedation is remarkably safe. However, if you have significant medical problems, sedation, like all forms of anesthesia, can be a stress to your system. A health evaluation and physical exam by your internist or primary care physician is important before surgery if you have significant medical problems.

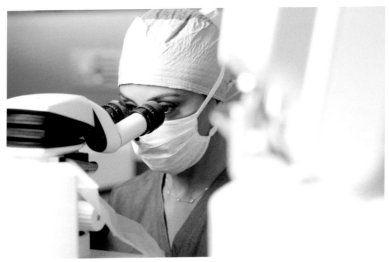

Dr. Shamie is shown using an operating microscope to perform cataract surgery. The procedure usually takes about ten minutes per eye to perform.

The purpose is to verify that you are healthy enough to receive sedation during the surgery, and that you're not having unexplained symptoms such as chest pain. If you have significant health issues, you will need to have a comprehensive health evaluation by your doctor within thirty days before surgery.

If you are healthy, an extra physical exam is almost certainly a waste of time and money. Nevertheless, as we write this, you still have to have a comprehensive health exam within thirty days before cataract surgery. This is a requirement made by the bureaucrats in Washington, DC, who are talented at increasing the cost of health care and decreasing its efficiency (but that is a subject for another book). What if you already had your annual checkup thirty-one days before surgery? Too bad—you have to do it again. There is a ray of hope. Our ophthalmology specialty societies are working to convince the bureaucrats to change the regulations. Hopefully by the time you read this, things will have changed. For now, though, everyone has to have a comprehensive general health evaluation within thirty days before surgery.

Three Days before Surgery

If you wear soft contact lenses, remove the lens from the eye to be treated and leave it out starting three days before the surgery. Hard lenses should be out for two weeks prior to surgery.

If you haven't yet done so, arrange for someone to drive you home after surgery and make sure you are okay at home. This is important, because you will not be able to drive right after surgery; you'll be a little groggy from the sedative, your pupil will be dilated, and your vision will be too blurry to drive.

The Night before Surgery

Don't have anything to eat or drink for six hours preceding your surgery, including water. It is important that your sedation be done on an empty stomach. If there is food in your stomach while you are sedated, you can burp it up and inhale it into your lungs accidentally. This can cause a serious pneumonia. For the same reason, don't have a giant meal six hours and one minute before surgery. Eat a light breakfast early if your surgery is in the afternoon. Note: you *should* take your routine prescription medications the morning of surgery, and it is fine to take the pills with small sips of water.

Clean off all makeup from your face and eyelids and eyelashes the night before. It is important that your face be very clean, so it can be properly disinfected at the surgery center.

The Day of Surgery

Don't wear makeup or fragrances, including scented lotions or hair products. Don't wear jewelry or other valuables—leave these at home. Do wear comfortable street clothes, including a shirt that buttons up the front. These are the clothes you'll be wearing during surgery, so make sure they're loose, not binding.

- Take your insurance card to the surgical center.
- Take a list of all your medications and any allergies.
- Arrive an hour before the scheduled time for surgery. Plan to be at the surgical center for about two and a half hours.

At the Surgical Center

A fully staffed operating room in a certified surgical center is the best environment for cataract surgery. High standards for cleanliness and the presence of a board-certified anesthesiologist can help ensure that there are no problems.

- The nursing staff will check your blood pressure and insert an intravenous (IV) line, which the anesthesiologist will use to administer the sedative.
- The surgery eye will be marked with an ink pen, so no one can possibly be confused about which eye is being done. You may notice the mark on your forehead after surgery.
- Cataract surgery is done with a dilated pupil. A nurse will put drops in your eye to numb the eye and dilate the pupil.

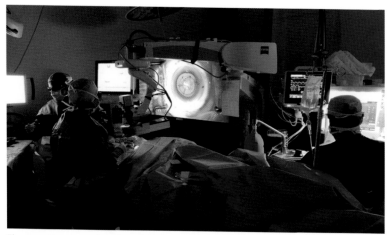

The operating room is a hive of activity. The surgeon is on the left with the scrub nurse behind him. The anesthesiologist is on the right. The eye appears on a TV monitor so everyone can follow the procedure.

- Heart monitors will be placed on your chest (this is why we recommend that you wear a front-buttoning shirt).

The Cataract Procedure

We described cataract surgery in detail in chapter 5. Here we focus on your experience of the surgery rather than the procedure itself.

- You'll lie on your back for the procedure. The staff will cover you with a blanket to keep you warm, and place neck and knee supports under you to make you comfortable. You will lie with your hands by your side. Don't raise your hands to touch or scratch your face. Your hands can carry germs into the sterile area.

- If you are undergoing laser cataract surgery, it is done first. You are given mild IV sedation and the laser treatment is performed. The actual treatment takes about ninety seconds.

- Next, for both manual and laser surgery, your eyelid, eyelashes, and face will be cleaned with an antibacterial iodine solution to eliminate as much as possible any possibility of infection. The iodine cleansing is just one of several ways of ensuring that the procedure is completely sanitary.

- Your face is completely covered with a special sterile sheet that has an opening over the eye. This keeps bacteria from your nose and mouth away from your eye.

- An air tube is placed beneath the sheet to release a gentle flow of oxygen toward your face. Some people worry that they won't be able to breathe because their face is covered, but there is no need to worry: you will get plenty of air.

- Your eye is completely numbed with eye drops.

- As these preparations are going on, the anesthesiologist is giving you more sedation through the IV line to ensure you are relaxed and comfortable. He or she will be sitting by your side the entire time, monitoring your vital signs throughout the procedure and keeping you sedated.

- The surgery is then done, as described in chapter 5. While you are sedated, you will notice lights and kaleidoscopic colors. You will not see instruments coming at your eye, nor can you see the procedure being performed.

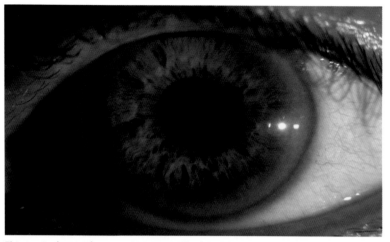

This eye is shown after cataract surgery. The lens implant is not visible—it sits behind the iris of the eye.

It's important to note that we don't try to put you to sleep for cataract surgery, although patients often do fall asleep. The sedation is designed to make you so relaxed that you don't care at all that someone is doing surgery on your eye. If you fall asleep, that is fine. If you are awake and happy, that is fine, too. If you start feeling any anxiety, say so. The anesthesiologist will immediately give you more sedation.

If the surgery is performed manually, the procedure itself takes about ten minutes. In a procedure performed with a laser, the procedure takes about ninety seconds. Thanks to the sedation, when it's over, the patient's reaction is usually, "What? It's over already? That was fast!"

Immediately after Your Surgery

In the recovery room, a nurse will check your blood pressure again, give you something to eat or drink, and monitor you for twenty minutes or so.

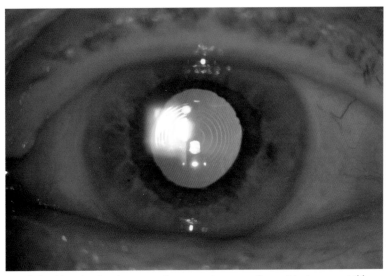

A multifocal lens implant in an eye after cataract surgery. Concentric rings are visible on the surface of the lens implant. These rings allow the multifocal lens to give both good distance and good near vision without glasses.

When you are awake and able to walk safely, you can be driven home. We recommend you take a nap. Your eyes will still be dilated and you will be light sensitive and have blurry vision for the rest of the day.

At home, use the prescribed eye drops as instructed, starting the day of surgery. You may notice scratchy irritation, like a grain of sand in your eye. This is generally gone by the next morning. Your eye may be somewhat sore. Feel free to take an over-the-counter pain reliever. You should *not* have strong pain in or around your eye. That is abnormal and can signify high pressure in your eye. If that happens, call your doctor immediately.

The Day after Surgery

You will wake up to clearer vision, but don't expect it to be perfect. You will need to go to your doctor's office for a short checkup. Feel free to drive yourself if you feel comfortable—usually vision is better the day after surgery than it was the day before. Don't be surprised if your pupil is still dilated the day after surgery. We use very strong dilating drops, which take 24 to 48 hours to wear off. Get a ride if you aren't sure you can drive safely. The doctor will check your eye pressure and be sure you are healing well with minimal inflammation.

The Week after Surgery

You can largely go back to your normal routine right away. We use very small incisions, so you can even exercise vigorously and lift heavy weights the next day. A week after surgery, your vision should be excellent, and it will usually improve a little more as you heal over the next few months. You can go back to your usual work and play, with a few exceptions:

- For the first five days, don't wear old eye makeup. If you use mascara or eyeliner, open a fresh tube. Old makeup can contain harmful bacteria.
- Use your eye drops according to your doctor's instructions. These are important to prevent infection and reduce inflammation.
- Stay out of swimming pools, hot tubs, Jacuzzis, steam baths, and saunas for a week. Showering and bathing are fine.
- Avoid rubbing your eye for the first week.

Now that you've been through the procedure, the next chapter talks about what to expect and the possible problems after surgery.

8

Risks, Side Effects, and Potential Complications

After your eyes have healed from the cataract surgery, your world will be brighter and clearer. You'll be able to focus better. You'll probably be amazed at how vivid colors appear—colors that faded as your cataracts grew. Contrast will be sharper. Ghosting and double vision will no longer be a problem.

You'll see well enough to work, to move around independently, and to enjoy the activities that you might have put on hold. If you have chosen an advanced lens, you'll be less dependent on eyeglasses—you might not need them at all. Cataract surgery isn't a fountain of youth, but it does improve your vision. Being in your sixties, seventies, eighties, or nineties, and having the vision of a forty-year-old, is an amazing thing in itself. Within twenty-four hours your eyesight will be markedly improved—so much so that you'll probably be eager to schedule surgery for the other eye at your follow-up visit to your doctor.

Have Realistic Expectations

No replacement lens, however sophisticated it might be, is as good as a young, healthy *natural lens.* Though your vision will almost certainly be better than before your surgery, it will not be as sharp as a teenager's. Nighttime halos and glare, double vision, and ghosting will be significantly better, but may not be eliminated altogether.

If you've chosen laser cataract surgery, the surgeon will usually plan to target you for excellent distance vision or monovision, with one eye focused for distance and the other eye for near. The choice is up to you. With an advanced lens, the surgeon will likely plan to give you an increased range of vision in each eye without glasses, minimizing the need for those annoying reading glasses perched on your nose or dangling around your neck.

Even with advanced lenses and laser cataract surgery, though, we still can't promise perfect vision. Everyone heals differently, which changes each person's result slightly. Expect to have very good vision but also expect that you may still wear glasses when you need perfect vision. Even so, instead of wearing glasses 90 percent of the time, you may only be wearing them 10 percent of the time, or even less. By having a clouded natural lens replaced with a clear, permanent, state-of-the-art synthetic lens, you will see images more vividly than you have for years. You'll enjoy greater independence for a wider range of activities with less dependence—maybe even no dependence—on eyeglasses.

Cataract surgery has amazing benefits and is also remarkably safe. Still, like all medical procedures, cataract surgery has possible risks and complications. We'll review these in detail in the rest of this chapter.

Normal Side Effects

There are a few minor side effects that are common. Mild aching is common for a few days, but it should be mild enough that Tylenol or ibuprofen can relieve it. Notify your doctor if you have moderate or worse aching in the first few days, or any aching after a week.

Your eye will be light sensitive the day of surgery because of the dilation. Mild light sensitivity can last a few days, but generally not longer. If you have light sensitivity after a few days, let your doctor know.

Also normal and to be expected are itching, scratchiness, and watering for a week. Your vision will fluctuate for a week as the incisions heal.

During Surgery: Potential Complications

Complications during surgery are quite rare when you're in the hands of an experienced surgeon, but they still can happen. The two most common problems during surgery are damage to the capsular bag and damage to the ligament that holds the new lens implant.

Occasionally, the process of removing the cataract can damage the capsular bag. In that case, the surgeon generally has to use a standard lens implant, even if you chose an advanced lens before surgery. This complication can also lead, after surgery, to swelling in the retina, which can blur your vision, or a retinal detachment. There is good evidence that laser cataract surgery reduces the risk of damage to the capsular bag, which is in part why we strongly prefer the laser.

Sometimes during surgery we discover that there is damage to the ligament, or zonule, that holds the new lens implant in place. This isn't really a complication, because the problem was there before surgery, but this condition makes surgery more difficult. A damaged ligament may not hold the new lens implant in the proper position. Sometimes suturing of the lens implant is required, and sometimes a different lens implant is used.

After Surgery: Potential Complications

There are a variety of possible complications after surgery, but fortunately most are minor or easily managed. A few do require emergency intervention. We review these here, so you'll be aware of what can go wrong and how to respond.

Posterior Capsule Opacification (After-Cataract)

When the clouded natural lens is removed and a synthetic lens implanted, it is impossible for the cataract to come back. Sometimes, however, the part of the capsular bag behind the new implant becomes cloudy. This causes blurry vision or glare because the light passing through the new lens implant is distorted by the opacity. This condition is called *posterior capsule opacification,* or, more colloquially, an *after-cataract.* It is quite common, affecting 30 percent of all cataract patients, and occurs from one month to many years after surgery.

Fortunately, the problem can be quickly and safely repaired with a three-minute outpatient procedure called *YAG laser capsulotomy.* Your surgeon will use a laser to make a small window in the back of the capsular bag, clearing the opacity away. The procedure is painless, requiring no incision or sutures.

Floaters

You'll see everything more clearly—including any preexisting *floaters,* those little objects in the vitreous humor that float across your field of vision. If you notice something that looks like a few gnats or strands flying across your field of vision when you move your eyes, it's nothing to be concerned about. If the floaters are bothersome, there are treatments for these—either a laser treatment to break up the floaters or a surgery to remove them entirely.

Retinal Detachment

In less than 1 percent of patients, vitreous fluid seeps through a tear in the retina after cataract surgery, separating the retina from the back of the eye. This is called a *retinal detachment.* Extremely nearsighted patients are at greater-than-normal risk for retinal detachment.

Often retinal detachments are preceded by a shower of new floaters, much like a swarm of gnats. While a few floaters are nothing to worry about, a burst of new floaters is concerning. Another symptom that can precede a retinal detachment is momentary flashes of light in your peripheral vision, akin to fireworks. If you have flashes, there is no need to panic, though. These are usually due to reflections of light from the new lens implant, and not the beginning of a retinal detachment.

You can tell the difference by going into a dark room. Flashes from the lens implant will disappear in a dark room, but flashes from the possible beginnings of a retinal detachment will persist in the dark. Either new floaters or flashes can be a harbinger of a retinal detachment—you should call your doctor. This is not an emergency, but typically the doctor will see you in the next few days.

The first symptom of a true retinal detachment is a curtain or dark area moving across the vision in one eye. If not treated promptly, it can progress to complete loss of vision. Retinal detachment is a medical emergency. If you have symptoms of darkness moving across your vision, you should seek treatment immediately, day or night, holiday or weekend. Fortunately, retinal detachments are almost always treatable with restoration of vision, but the quicker it is treated, the better the vision will recover.

Inflammation

Mild inflammation within the eye is normal for a few weeks after surgery. You will take anti-inflammatory drops to suppress this. Sometimes when the drops are discontinued, after a month or so, inflammation can return. Your eye will be mildly red, achy, and possibly light sensitive. If you have these symptoms, return to the doctor to get more anti-inflammatory drops.

Cystoid Macular Edema

Sometimes inflammation after surgery can affect the retina. This condition, called *cystoid macular edema,* causes fluid accumulation in the macula. Since the macula is the part of the eye responsible for *central vision,* this can cause significantly blurry vision. Cystoid macular edema is usually easily controlled with anti-inflammatory eye drops, but sometimes stronger medicines or implants are required. The risk of this problem is minimized by making sure that all remnants of the cataract are thoroughly removed during surgery. It is one of the ways in which a skilled surgeon can achieve better results for you.

Infection

The rarest form of inflammation after cataract surgery is caused by infection. Fewer than one-tenth of 1 percent (0.1 percent) of cataract surgery patients get *endophthalmitis,* a bacterial (or occasionally fungal) infection of the inside of the eye. Symptoms can include moderate aching pain, loss of vision, and light sensitivity. Typically, endophthalmitis starts two to four days after surgery. If not treated immediately, the infection can cause permanent impairment of vision. The usual treatment is injection of antibiotics into the eye. Sometimes *vitrectomy*—removal of the vitreous—is necessary to control the infection. If you have these symptoms you should contact your doctor immediately. As long as the infection is caught early, vision can usually be saved.

Corneal Edema

The inner layer, or endothelium, of the cornea is a layer of cells that keep fluid from accumulating in the cornea. When this layer is damaged, fluid builds up, causing blurry vision. This problem usually only happens if you have a preexisting disease of the endothelium, called Fuchs' dystrophy. The surgeon will explain this to you ahead of time. Rarely, *corneal edema* can result unexpectedly from a complicated cataract surgery. It often goes away on its own, but if not you may need a partial corneal transplant to cure the problem. This is another case where surgeon experience makes the operation safer.

Unstable Lens Implant

Rarely, the implanted lens shifts or rotates within the eye. This can cause double vision, ghost images, or blurry vision. This problem can usually be corrected with glasses, but sometimes another surgery is needed to reposition or replace the implant.

Incorrect Prescription

A capable, experienced eye surgeon will carefully calculate the power for your new lens implant using measurements of the cornea and the length of the eye. This calculation is less accurate if you are extremely farsighted or nearsighted or if you've had LASIK previously. Even the most experienced surgeon occasionally has a patient turn out significantly more nearsighted or farsighted than expected. We call this a refractive surprise. Believe us: it is just as surprising to us as it is to the patient. The solution is to perform laser surgery to correct the refractive error, or to replace the lens implant with one of the appropriate power.

When to Call Your Doctor

Trust your intuition. If you feel something is seriously wrong, contact your surgeon right away, even if it is the middle of the night. Your surgeon must have someone available for emergency coverage 24/7/365. Symptoms to worry about are moderate or severe aching pain in or around your eye, moderate or severe light sensitivity, or a significant increase in redness. Loss of vision, significant worsening of vision, or a dark area in your vision are all causes for concern.

Get in touch with your doctor right away or follow his or her emergency instructions. Almost anything that goes wrong after cataract surgery can be successfully cured if treated properly and promptly.

9

The Future of Cataract Treatment

As America ages, the volume of cataract surgery is skyrocketing, as is the demand for even greater safety, convenience, and clarity of vision. Researchers throughout the world are investigating, testing, or introducing lens materials, surgical techniques, and prevention methods that could revolutionize the treatment not only of cataracts but also other eye conditions, such as glaucoma, macular degeneration, and presbyopia. Here are some of the most exciting new developments.

New Lens Implants

The hottest area of innovation is in new lens implants to give better vision without glasses.

Accommodating Lens Implants

Accommodating lenses are designed to mimic the movement of the natural lens to allow you to see far away and up close. One accommodating lens, the Crystalens, is already available (*see* chapter 5). Unfortunately, the Crystalens doesn't give much accommodation, and therefore isn't often used, so alternatives are under investigation. The alternatives designs are mechanical and electro-optical.

The mechanical designs rely on a tiny muscle, called the *ciliary muscle,* that surrounds the equator of your natural lens. This muscle normally controls accommodation, the process of focusing your eye from distance to near. These designs use the ciliary muscle to pump fluid in or out of the center of the lens when you focus for near or distance. These lenses in theory can allow for excellent distance and near vision. These lenses are still being perfected, and are not yet available anywhere in the world. Unfortunately, it seems to us that these lenses won't give accurate corrections, so you will likely still need distance glasses.

Electro-optical lenses may solve this problem. These lenses will have a tiny battery and microchip that adjust the power of the lens for near or far, providing excellent vision at both distances. These designs are still theoretical, and inventors are trying to figure out how to recharge the battery. We think these lenses are a decade or more from being available.

Glaucoma and Cataract Surgery

Glaucoma means that you have too much pressure in your eye, akin to elevated blood pressure. Over many years, the pressure can damage the nerve in your eye, causing vision loss. One longtime treatment for glaucoma is creating a drainage path, so excessive pressure can flow out of the eye. This has been an area of active innovation. Already, several products are available that can be combined with cataract surgery to lower eye pressure. One is a stent that props open the eye's natural drainage channel. Others allow the surgeon to create a tiny hole from the inside of the eye outward to drain fluid. More options will become available in the next few years.

Also Being Studied

- Development of an injectable gel that can fill the capsular bag and solidify after the cataract is removed. This gel hardens into a lens after injection. This would eliminate the need for a lens implant, and ideally would focus for both distance and near, like the natural lens of a young person.
- Genetic research that could lead to gene therapy for cataracts and other eye disorders.
- Treatment of the rare cataracts that occur in babies by regrowing a natural lens.
- An implant that slowly releases drugs that can be placed in the eye at the end of surgery so that eye drops are not necessary.

Ophthalmic researchers and optical scientists envision exciting possibilities for safe, noninvasive ways to prevent and correct vision damage in people of all ages. Some of the developments described above are many years away from practical application. Others are just becoming available for use by experienced eye surgeons.

One thing is certain: cataract surgery and lens replacement have made huge strides in just the past few years. Barely fifty years ago, patients spent two weeks in the hospital after cataract surgery, lying on their back with sandbags on either side of their head to keep them from moving. There were no lens implants, so patients had to wear Coke-bottle glasses permanently. Now, the procedure takes ten minutes. You leave for home twenty minutes later, and you are back to normal activity the next day.

If you elect to have advanced cataract surgery, you likely will have excellent vision with no need for glasses at all. The procedure is safer and faster, and the results more satisfying, than anyone could have imagined in the days of sandbags and hospitals. If you have cataract surgery today, you can thank the pioneering work of scientists and eye specialists for restored clarity of vision, independence, and quality of life that you will appreciate as never before.

Resources

The below websites provide additional resources you may find helpful in learning more about key topics covered in this book including the steps of cataract surgery, advanced lenses, and choosing a surgeon, among others. Within each site is an internal search bar in the header. Search for "cataract surgery" to explore their objectively written cataract content.

The editorial information provided on these sites are not intended to be a substitute for professional medical advice, diagnosis, or treatment. Always seek the advice of your physician or other qualified health provider with any questions you may have regarding cataract diagnosis and surgery.

American Academy of Ophthalmology (AAO)
www.aao.org/eye-health/diseases/what-are-cataracts

All About Vision
www.allaboutvision.com/conditions/cataracts.htm

MedicineNet
www.medicinenet.com/cataract_surgery/article.htm

WebMD
www.webmd.com/eye-health/cataracts/what-are-cataracts#1

Glossary

Numbers

20/20 vision: Normal visual acuity. The numbers indicate that the tested eye, 20 feet away from the eye chart, sees as well as a person with normal vision at the same distance.

A

ablation: Removal or vaporization of tissue with a laser.

accommodating lens: A lens implant that enables the patient to change his or her focus from distance to near without reading glasses by changing its power in response to contractions of the ciliary muscle.

accommodation: The eye's ability to change the shape of the natural lens, by contraction of the ciliary muscle, in order to focus clearly on objects up close. As the natural lens becomes more rigid with age—a condition called *presbyopia*—it is less able to accommodate, so reading glasses are needed.

after-cataract: *See* posterior capsule opacification.

amblyopia: Also called *lazy eye*, amblyopia is poor vision, usually in one eye but occasionally in both eyes, that develops in the first five years of life. It is caused by suppression of vision in the affected eye, which impairs the development of visual pathways from the eye to the brain.

anterior chamber: Space between the cornea and the iris. It is filled with fluid called aqueous humor.

aqueous humor: Clear, watery fluid that fills the anterior chamber of the eye. It maintains intraocular pressure and nourishes the cornea, iris, and natural lens.

astigmatism: Visual distortion caused by a cornea whose surface is elongated like the side of a football rather than round like a basketball. Light rays enter the eye unequally and produce two focal points on the retina.

B

biometry: Measurement of the length of the eye.

biomicroscope: *See* slit lamp.

C

capsule or capsular bag: A thin membrane that forms the outermost layer of the natural lens. It surrounds the cortex and the nucleus.

capsulorhexis: A hole made in the front part of the capsular bag during cataract surgery to allow removal of the underlying cortex and nucleus. The new lens implant is inserted through the capsulorhexis to center inside the capsular bag.

capsulotomy: *See* YAG laser capsulotomy.

cataract: Clouded area or opacity of the eye's natural lens. Cataracts are usually caused by aging, but can be congenital or caused by trauma, disease, or high-dose steroid use.

central vision: The area around whatever thing you are looking at, in contrast to peripheral vision. This is the sharpest area of vision, and it used to distinguish detail and color. The macula is the part of the retina that is responsible for central vision.

ciliary muscle: A tiny muscle that surrounds the eye's natural lens, and contracts or relaxes, thereby changing the shape of the natural lens and allowing it to focus on objects both close up and far away.

cone: One of more than 7 million retinal photoreceptor cells (in each eye) concentrated in the macular area of the retina, responsible for sharp vision and the ability to see colors.

congenital cataract: A cataract that is present at birth.

conjunctiva: Clear mucous membrane that covers the white of the eye (sclera) and lines the inner surface of the eyelids.

cornea: Clear, curved protrusion at the front of the eye through which light first passes. Contact lenses sit on the cornea. The cornea covers and protects the iris, pupil, and anterior chamber.

corneal edema: Abnormal fluid buildup in the cornea, which consequently causes swelling and blurred vision.

corneal topography: A precise three-dimensional map of the cornea using sophisticated camera and computer technology.

cortex: Soft, clear tissue that forms the middle layer of the eye's natural lens, between the capsular bag and the nucleus.

cortical cataract: A cataract that begins as whitish, wedge-shaped opaque areas in the lens cortex, eventually becoming streaks reaching inward to the center of the natural lens, like spokes on a wheel.

Crystalens: an artificial lens used to treat cataracts. It is not often used because its ability to accommodate is limited.

cystoid macular edema: A condition in which fluid-filled cysts develop in the macula, causing retinal swelling and blurred vision. A complication of cataract surgery that typically resolves with anti-inflammatory eye drops.

D

diabetes: More properly called *diabetes mellitus,* a disease in which there is an excessive amount of sugar in the bloodstream. People with diabetes can develop retina problems, and are more likely to develop cystoid macular edema after cataract surgery.

double vision: The condition in which two images of a single object are seen. Double vision can be *binocular,* caused by the eyes not working together. Binocular double vision disappears when either eye is covered, and is caused by strabismus. Double vision can also be *monocular,* which means it persists when one eye is covered. Monocular double vision is common with cataracts. *See also* ghost image.

E

endophthalmitis: A serious infection, usually caused by bacteria, of the interior of the eye.

extended-depth-of-focus (EDOF) lens: *See* extended-range lens.

extended-range lens: An advanced lens implant that provides a greater range of vision by stretching out the point of best focus. These implants give good vision from far distance to about 28 inches away.

F

farsightedness: *See* hyperopia.

femtosecond laser: A cold laser with ultrashort pulses that is used to cut tissue precisely. *See* laser cataract surgery.

field of vision: *See* visual field.

floaters: Particles that drift around in the vitreous humor. People see these as dots or lines in their vision, particularly when looking at a blank background. They can be annoying.

free radical: An atom, usually oxygen, that has an unpaired electron, making the atom likely to react with other molecules and damage them.

G

ghost image: Distortion of vision similar to double vision. With double vision, however, you'll see two relatively clear images, whereas a ghost image is a faint copy that appears next to the object you are looking at. Cataracts commonly cause ghost images.

glare: Sensation of dazzling, intense, scattered light when looking at a light source; often due to cataracts. Glare is most noticeable at night looking at headlights or streetlights.

glaucoma: A disease that damages the nerve of the eye, usually because the intraocular pressure is too high. If untreated, glaucoma can lead to blindness.

H

halo: Perceived rings around light sources viewed at night; often accompanied by glare. Halos are a common symptom of cataracts, but can also occur after cataract surgery, although usually to a lesser degree.

haptics: The side struts on a lens implant that help to hold it centered in the capsular bag after implantation.

hypermature cataract: A cataract that is so far advanced it is causing inflammation or glaucoma in the affected eye.

hyperopia: Also called *farsightedness,* hyperopia occurs when the eye is too short and images come into focus behind the retina. A farsighted person finds that close vision is very blurry and distance vision is often blurry as well.

I

immature cataract: A cataract that is not well advanced, cannot be seen with the naked eye, and may not yet interfere significantly with vision.

intraocular lens: *See* lens implant.

intraocular pressure: Fluid pressure within the eye. The intraocular pressure is normally between 10 and 21 mmHg.

IOL: *See* lens implant.

iris: The colored ring in the visible eye. The pupil is a hole in the center of the iris that allows light to enter the eye.

L

laser cataract surgery: Use of the femtosecond laser to create a perfectly circular capsulorhexis and to break up the nucleus for easy and nontraumatic removal. The laser can also be used at the same time to create limbal-relaxing incisions to correct astigmatism.

LASIK: Acronym for LAser *In-situ* Keratomileusis, a laser procedure that reshapes the cornea to correct nearsightedness, farsightedness, and astigmatism.

lazy eye: *See* amblyopia.

legally blind: Having vision of 20/200 or worse, even with an optimal pair of glasses.

lens: *See* lens implant; natural lens.

lens implant: A synthetic lens implanted during cataract surgery to replace the natural lens. Officially it is called an *intraocular lens,* or *IOL.* Lens implants are made of soft silicone or acrylic material.

limbal-relaxing incisions: An astigmatism-management technique that involves making a pair of small incisions in the cornea near the limbus. These incisions cause the cornea to relax into a rounder shape, correcting the astigmatism.

limbus: The junction between the cornea and the sclera. Seen in a mirror, the limbus appears to be a gray area between the colored and the white part of the eye.

M

macula: The small central area of the retina filled with cone photoreceptors that is responsible for providing sharp central vision.

macular degeneration: A progressive eye disease caused by age-related deterioration of the macula.

mature cataract: A cataract that has advanced to the point where the natural lens appears milky.

monofocal lens: A basic lens implant that is similar to a disposable camera lens, in that it has a single fixed focal point, usually designed for mid-distance vision. Eyeglasses are needed for good vision at other distances.

monovision: Having one eye focused for distance vision and the other for near vision. Monovision is an effective treatment for presbyopia (the loss of reading vision with age), but not all people can tolerate the imbalance between the eyes.

multifocal lens implant: An advanced lens implant that has two or more focal points. It is designed to provide good near, midrange, and distance vision without glasses. A multifocal lens implant is not quite as sharp for distance as the other implants.

myopia: Also called *nearsightedness,* this occurs when the eye is "too long" and images come into focus before they reach the retina. A nearsighted person can see close objects clearly but has difficulty seeing objects at a distance.

N

natural lens: The lens you were born with. It is a clear, flexible lens made of proteins called crystallines. It is located behind the iris, and focuses rays of light onto the retina. In young people it is soft enough to respond to contractions of the ciliary muscle by changing shape, allowing for good close vision. With age it hardens, causing presbyopia.

nearsightedness: *See* myopia.

nuclear cataract: Clouding of the nucleus of the lens due to aging or high myopia.

nucleus: The firm center, or core, of the natural lens, surrounded by the cortex, which in turn is surrounded by the capsular bag.

O

ophthalmologist: A medical doctor who specializes in the medical and surgical treatment of eye disease.

ophthalmoscope: An illuminated instrument using mirrors to examine the retina and macula.

optic nerve: A bundle of nerve fibers that transmit visual impulses from the retina to the brain. It can be damaged in eyes with glaucoma.

optician: One who is trained to fit and dispense eyeglasses and, in some U.S. states, contact lenses, according to a prescription from an optometrist or ophthalmologist. Outside the United States, some countries license opticians to do eye exams.

optometrist: An eye doctor who provides general eye care, and is qualified to diagnose and treat vision disorders not requiring specialized medical or surgical intervention.

P

perimeter: A device that emits flashes of light to test the visual field and peripheral vision. It reveals blind spots, which can be a sign of glaucoma.

peripheral vision: Side vision; your ability to see objects and movement that you aren't directly looking at. *See also* central vision.

phacoemulsification: Surgical procedure to remove a cataract using ultrasound to break up the lens, the pieces of which are then removed by suction. Laser cataract surgery uses a laser to break up the lens.

phoropter: An eye testing device consisting of a complete range of corrective lenses that can be adjusted to hundreds of combinations. The patient is asked to evaluate by answering, "Which is better, one or two?" By continually changing the lenses, the doctor can arrive at a combination of lens strengths that becomes the basis of a prescription for corrective lenses.

photoreceptors: Light-sensitive cells—rods and cones—in the retina that allow the eye to see in dim light, distinguish colors, and perceive contrast.

posterior capsule: The back part of the capsular bag, which is left in place during cataract surgery to help support the new lens implant. A posterior capsule tear is one of the complications of cataract surgery that is made less likely by performing laser cataract surgery.

posterior capsule opacification: An opacity that can develop on the posterior capsule at any time after cataract surgery. It causes blurry vision, and is easily treated with YAG laser capsulotomy.

posterior chamber: The fluid-filled area between the iris and the lens.

posterior subcapsular cataract: A cataract that begins at the back of the lens, on the back surface of the capsular bag.

potential acuity testing: Pre-surgical assessment of a patient's likely visual acuity if the cataract is removed, using a special device that projects light through the cataract onto the retina.

presbyopia: Loss of sharpness in close vision caused by age-related stiffening of the natural lens and accompanying reduction in ability to accommodate.

pupil: The circular opening in the center of the iris. Through contraction or expansion of the iris, the pupil shrinks or grows to regulate the amount of light that enters the eye.

R

refraction: Bending of light as it passes from one material to another. Also, a test to determine the eye's refractive error.

refractive error: Optical defect producing blurred vision due to light rays not converging precisely on the retina. The refractive error can be nearsightedness, farsightedness, or astigmatism.

refractive surgery: A surgical procedure to correct the eye's refractive error, such as LASIK. LASIK or other procedures can be done after cataract surgery if you find you still need glasses for excellent distance vision.

retina: A smooth, thin layer of tissue at the back of the eye, containing photoreceptor cells, which convert reflected light into electrical impulses that move along the optic nerve to the brain.

retinal detachment: Separation of the retina from the underlying tissue, requiring urgent surgery to prevent blindness.

ripe cataract: *See* mature cataract.

rod: One of more than 120 million retinal photoreceptor cells (in each eye) that are especially receptive to brightness and allow us to see in very dim light.

S

sclera: An opaque, fibrous, protective covering that surrounds the eye. It is the white part of the eye.

second sight: A temporary, cataract-induced improvement in vision among farsighted people, usually associated with nuclear cataracts.

slit lamp: A microscope that projects a flattened beam of light into the eye for close examination of internal structures. The slit lamp is the primary instrument for diagnosing cataracts

Snellen chart: The standard tool to measure visual acuity, this is a chart consisting of rows of letters with the largest letters at the top and the smallest at the bottom. It was developed by Dutch ophthalmologist Hermann Snellen in 1862. It is usually read at a distance of 20 feet, which gives us the 20/20 notation for visual acuity.

steroid: A drug, often a type of hormone, that is prescribed to relieve swelling and inflammation.

strabismus: An eye misalignment caused by an imbalance in muscles that move the eyeballs. People with strabismus are sometimes referred to as "cross-eyed" or "wall-eyed." The eyes can turn inward or outward, or one eye can point higher than the other. Strabismus is a common cause of double vision.

subcapsular cataract: *See* posterior subcapsular cataract.

T

tonometer: An instrument that measures intraocular pressure. It is used in the diagnosis of glaucoma.

tonometry: Measurement of intraocular pressure with a tonometer.

toric lens: An advanced lens implant designed to correct astigmatism. Other types of advanced implants can also include the toric feature to correct astigmatism. For example, there are toric accommodating lenses and toric extended range lenses.

traumatic cataract: A cataract that is caused by direct blow to the eye.

U

ultraviolet (UV) radiation: Electromagnetic radiation, shorter in wavelength than visible radiation but longer than X-rays. Ultraviolet rays may contribute to cataract development.

V

visual acuity: Sharpness of vision. Visual acuity is measured on a Snellen chart.

visual field: The area of the world visible to an eye looking straight ahead; includes central vision and peripheral vision.

vitrectomy: Surgical removal of the vitreous humor, which is replaced with clear fluid. Vitrectomy is used to treat retinal detachment or to eliminate floaters.

vitreous or vitreous humor: A clear gel-like substance that fills the eye behind the natural lens and in front of the retina.

Y

YAG laser capsulotomy: Surgery using an yttrium-aluminum-garnet (YAG) laser is used to open a window in the posterior capsule, which eliminates posterior capsule opacification and clears up blurry vision.

Z

zonule: The circular ligament that attaches the natural lens to the ciliary muscle. Contraction and relaxation of the ciliary muscle is transmitted via the zonule to the natural lens, changing its shape. This allows the youthful eye to change its focus from far to near. The zonule also holds the capsular bag in place after cataract surgery, and thereby supports the new lens implant.

Index

Index

About the Authors

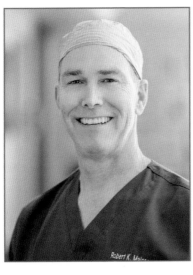

Robert K. Maloney, M.D., M.A. (Oxon), is managing partner of the Maloney-Shamie Vision Institute in West Los Angeles, California. Dr. Maloney was the first eye surgeon in western North America to perform LASIK surgery, as part of the original FDA clinical trials. Dr. Maloney has trained more than 1,000 surgeons in the use of the excimer laser and has personally performed more than 65,000 vision correction surgeries. He was voted by his peers one of America's top ten vision correction specialists in a nationwide survey conducted by *Ophthalmology Times.*

Dr. Maloney is a former Rhodes scholar and summa cum laude graduate of Harvard University. He is the recipient of the prestigious Lans Distinguished Award, given annually by the International Society of Refractive Surgery to one surgeon in the world for innovative contributions to the field of vision correction surgery.

Dr. Maloney holds eight patents. He is the author of four books and more than 175 articles, abstracts, and reports in professional journals. He has delivered more than 400 lectures on five continents to professional audiences. He has been a principal investigator for twenty FDA clinical trials.

Dr. Maloney has appeared frequently on television as the LASIK surgeon for the ABC hit series *Extreme Makeover.* He has appeared on the Discovery Channel, the Learning Channel, NBC, ABC, PBS, and CNN. He has also been featured in numerous magazines and newspapers.

He is married to Nicole Miller Maloney, a photographic artist. They have three children.

Dr. Maloney may be reached at the Maloney-Shamie Vision Institute at (310) 208-3937, or at **www.maloneyshamie.com.**

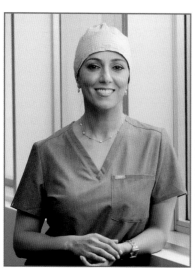

Neda Shamie, M.D., is a renowned LASIK, cataract, and corneal surgeon, and partner of the Maloney-Shamie Vision Institute in West Los Angeles, California. She previously was the medical director of the Doheny Eye Institute and is an adjunct clinical associate professor of ophthalmology at the Keck School of Medicine of USC.

Dr. Shamie graduated summa cum laude from UCLA and obtained her medical degree from UCSF School of Medicine. She completed her residency and fellowship training in corneal and laser refractive surgery at UC Irvine where she also served as director of the corneal service. Soon thereafter she joined the Devers Eye Institute in Portland, Oregon, where together with Dr. Mark Terry, she spearheaded many projects and advances in the field of lamellar corneal transplantation with emphasis on endothelial keratoplasty (DSEK and DMEK).

Dr. Shamie was the first surgeon in the Northwest to offer both artificial corneal transplantation and DMEK surgery to her patients. Recognized as an expert in complex vision correction surgery, Dr. Shamie has coauthored over fifty publications on the topics of cataract surgery and corneal transplantation, written eight chapters for surgical textbooks, and has led international lectures, courses, and seminars teaching colleagues about the advances in vision correction surgery. In 2017, the American Academy of Ophthalmology awarded her the Senior Achievement Award for contributions to the education of other eye surgeons. She has trained and instructed over 500 surgeons and has personally performed over 6,500 vision correction surgeries.

She is an active member of numerous ophthalmic societies, has served on the Cornea Clinical Committee of the American Society of Cataract and Refractive Surgery, was the president of the Los Angeles Society of Ophthalmology, and has been voted by peers to be among America's Top Doctors.

Dr. Shamie has two young daughters and is married to her college sweetheart, Sia Daneshmand, who is the head of Urologic Oncology at USC. In her spare time, she loves to travel to new destinations and create lasting memories with her family and friends.

Dr. Shamie may be reached at the Maloney-Shamie Vision Institute at (310) 208-3937, or at **www.maloneyshamie.com.**